D0404481

# Home Spa

# Home Spa

CREATING YOUR
OWN **SPA EXPERIENCE**
WITH AROMATHERAPY

JUDITH WHITE

**HAY HOUSE, INC.**
Carlsbad, California
London • Sydney • Johannesburg
Vancouver • Hong Kong • New Delhi

Copyright © 2006 by Judith White

**Published and distributed in the United States by:** Hay House, Inc.: www.hayhouse.com • **Published and distributed in Australia by:** Hay House Australia Pty. Ltd.: www.hayhouse.com.au • **Published and distributed in the United Kingdom by:** Hay House UK, Ltd.: www.hayhouse.co.uk • **Published and distributed in the Republic of South Africa by:** Hay House SA (Pty), Ltd.: orders@psdprom.co.za • **Distributed in Canada by:** Raincoast: www.raincoast.com • **Published in India by:** Hay House Publications (India) Pvt. Ltd.: www.hayhouseindia.co.in

*Designed by:* Rhett Nacson • *Edited by:* Rachel Eldred, Hay House Australia

All rights reserved. No part of this book may be reproduced by any mechanical, photographic, or electronic process, or in the form of a phonographic recording; nor may it be stored in a retrieval system, transmitted, or otherwise be copied for public or private use—other than for "fair use" as brief quotations embodied in articles and reviews—without prior written permission of the publisher.

The author of this book does not dispense medical advice or prescribe the use of any technique as a form of treatment for physical, emotional, or medical problems without the advice of a physician, either directly or indirectly. The intent of the author is only to offer information of a general nature to help you in your quest for emotional and spiritual well-being. In the event you use any of the information in this book for yourself, which is your constitutional right, the author and the publisher assume no responsibility for your actions.

**Library of Congress Control Number:** 2005935413

ISBN: 978-1-4019-1148-5

10  09  08  07    4  3  2  1
1st edition, January 2007

Printed in the United States of America

# contents

# Introduction

Humans love to be pampered, and in the 21st century the health spa has become not only the ultimate place to indulge, but the perfect place to relax – and it also assists you in maintaining good health. Unfortunately, for many of us, a visit to a spa is either a rare treat or a one-time rescue remedy.

Yet it needn't be: not if you create a spa environment at home. For most people, life is busy and it's difficult to find the time to rest and rejuvenate, but it isn't *that* difficult to create a mini-spa environment at home that you can enjoy every day. Even if it's for 10 minutes – enough time to soak your feet in an aromatic foot bath or give yourself a scentual shower. That's not difficult; the only requirements are the appropriate ingredients and techniques, which I shall provide in the chapters that follow.

My background and expertise is as an aromatherapist. I started work in the field in the 1980s when most people had no idea what an essential oil was, let alone what to do with it. Today it's different, and aromatherapy has become so widespread that you can pick up an essential oil in almost every health food store or pharmacy anywhere in the Western world. Aromatherapy is very popular in health spas, and to create your mini-spa at home you can use essential oils to not only set the scene but also to add to the many wonderful spa treatments that help rejuvenate body and soul – for example, foot soaks, body massages and facials.

It was my love of essential oils that inspired me to write this book; simply through the use of the oils in my day-to-day life, I had unwittingly created a mini-spa environment in my own home. They've touched every aspect of my life, and also allowed me to appreciate every moment of it. Ultimately, the creation of a home spa is simple: Take the time to truly be with and pamper yourself – even if it's for two or three minutes a day in a shower.

*Home Spa* is about encouraging you to maintain good health. It's about adopting a proactive role in your personal health and wellbeing. Like anything you value and care for, when you treat it well it responds favourably and, conversely, when you mistreat it, it can create havoc. So given that most of us want our body to be in optimum good health, the creation of a mini-spa environment at home is ideal.

## how to **use this** book

Simplicity is the key to *Home Spa*. The idea is to inspire you to create a mini-spa environment at home without too much fuss. The idea isn't to increase your workload, but rather lighten it. Chapter 1 starts with a brief overview on what spas are and how vital they are in today's world, while Chapter 2 provides tips on how to set the scene for your mini-spa environment at home. Chapter 3 provides a brief overview on the value of essential oils and how they work, and Chapter 4 gives a comprehensive profile on 26 essential oils as an easy reference source if you wish to treat specific ailments or concerns. You can refer to this chapter whenever you need specific information on an oil, but please remember to use your own intuition when you work with the oils – it's your own unique relationship with them that is of ultimate importance, as it inspires self-knowledge. Chapter 5 introduces many different spa techniques you can use in the comfort of your own home, from self-massage and sensual baths to aromatic footbaths and facials. Get ready to pamper yourself.

It takes 28 days to create a habit. In Chapter 6, I introduce you to the 28-Day Refocus Program. The simple tips I give are easy to incorporate into your everyday life – and so make it a daily habit. It needn't consume too much of your time, or distract you from your everyday tasks. On the contrary, it should assist you in decreasing stress levels so you get much more from your day.

My objective isn't to create a mini-spa environment at home to rival the health spa, but rather to complement it. A health spa is tremendously pampering and healing. Unfortunately, the healing experience often ends soon after you leave. The benefit of a mini-spa at home is that it prolongs your health spa experiences and assists you in keeping an equilibrium between spa visits – and it's that equilibrium that can assist you in dealing more effectively with the rigours of life.

*Home Spa* inspires a self-loving practice. When you rub your fingers and hands over your body with an essential oil blend you've created, you do more than just moisturise and protect the skin. You improve your circulation, tone the muscles and boost your immune system. The aromatic molecules can also help you to focus your thoughts and alter your mood as you spend quality time with yourself.

Ultimately, *Home Spa* is a guidebook – you won't just read it once, put it on your shelf and never look at it again. It shall be a constant point of reference as you define, and then continue to refine, your mini-spa experience at home.

When you take responsibility for your own health and wellbeing, your experience of life changes. You are not a victim of circumstance, but rather more powerful – you know and trust that you can take care of yourself no matter what life throws your way. *Home Spa* encourages you to do that. It invites you to make the most of your life, whatever it happens to present you with.

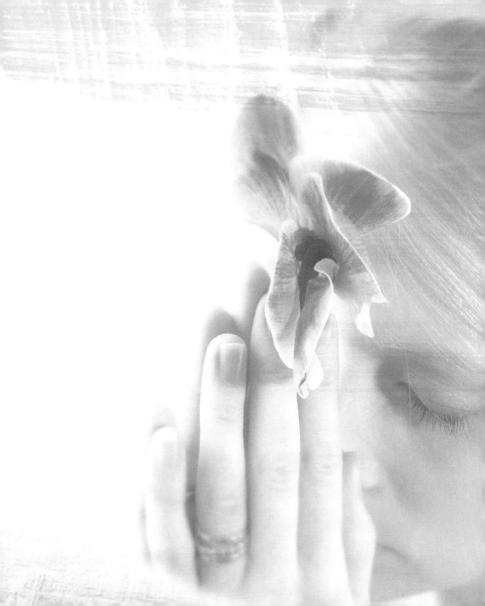

# chapter 1

## the beauty of spas

It wasn't that long ago when spas were simply thought of as pools of water with bubbles. Not anymore. Today, the spa is your one-stop health and pamper spot, and they've bred, it seems, in response to the busy-ness and demands of modern life. Since 1997 health spas in Australia have grown from a mere three to over three hundred.

As I mentioned in the introduction, your home mini-spa is to *complement* your visits to a health, or day, spa. The idea is to inspire you to keep abreast of lifestyle changes, as we know how easy it is to slip into self neglect when caught up in the busy-ness of life.

Good health in the 21st century is not simply the absence of disease; good health means you're on top of life … you feel great, you have the energy you need to get through the day, you are resilient to stress, your attitude to life is positive and you enjoy a healthy body weight. If this is not where you're at right now, it can be. Your visits to a spa, plus your own home mini-spa can help you achieve and sustain good health, so you meet the world with strength, character and determination.

But what is a spa and what can it offer? Each spa is unique in its own way. Some spas are big on hydrotherapy, others on health and nutrition. Some spas offer fitness regimes, while others focus on beauty treatments. For example, your local beauty salon may refer to itself as a spa simply because it offers massage. Essentially, though, today's modern spa is a health, beauty and fitness centre. And though massage is a treatment offered at most spa centres, at some you may also get nutritional and dietary advice and recommendations on how to change your lifestyle.

Health spas or resorts generally offer the more extensive options (along with the massage and pamper treats): Week-long health programs that focus on a specific issue such as weight loss; dietary and nutritional information; naturopathic and/or homeopathic advice; fitness and outdoor sports such as tennis; healthy gourmet cuisine; yoga and tai chi ... a visit every two years or so is the perfect way to keep on top of good health. In contrast, the day spa – as the name suggests – is a place to escape to for a day, or a few hours at least, where you get to relax and unwind with a number of pamper options: Massage, spa and sauna, facials, skin care treatments, hair care treatments, body rubs and scrubs, mud wraps, pedicures, manicures … some even offer more specialised treatments such as my very own crystal point therapy.

The distinction between the health spa and the day spa is general; ultimately, every spa is unique and there's no end to what a spa can offer. What is universal about the spa is its focus on the whole person; it inspires you to take care of your physical self (the body), your emotional self (most notably your stress levels which directly affect your body) and your spiritual self (you learn techniques on how to relax and let go of the concerns of the everyday, physical world). It's the ultimate place to nurture and care for yourself. You notice it as soon as you step through the doors: The gentle lights, the subtle scent of essential oils and other natural products, the sounds of water or gentle music. It's a haven for your soul, and a necessity in today's world to help us counteract the stress of modern life.

Ultimately, it's your ability to keep on top of things that determines your success in the world. That's not to suggest that we must behave like automated robots to get through life, it's simply to say that the more you look after and care for yourself (meet your needs) the more functional you can be in the world. It means that when things get difficult and you have challenges to face, you can remain calm. Rather than let the external circumstances affect you, you simply see them for what they are, deal with them as appropriately as you can and move on. That's what happens when we stop and take the time to look after ourselves, and that's the beauty of spas – they allow us to do that. They promote good health and a good mental attitude, which can help counter the often negative, self-limiting messages that we can be bombarded with every day.

Unfortunately, it's either impractical and/or costs too much to attend a spa too often. And that's why I suggest you set up a mini-spa at home. It's as simple as adding a few drops of essential oil to a bath.

Simple, with the promise of many added health benefits? Let's get started.

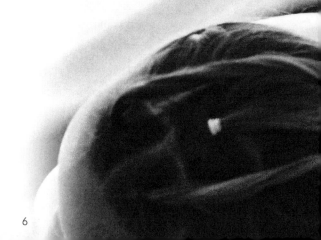

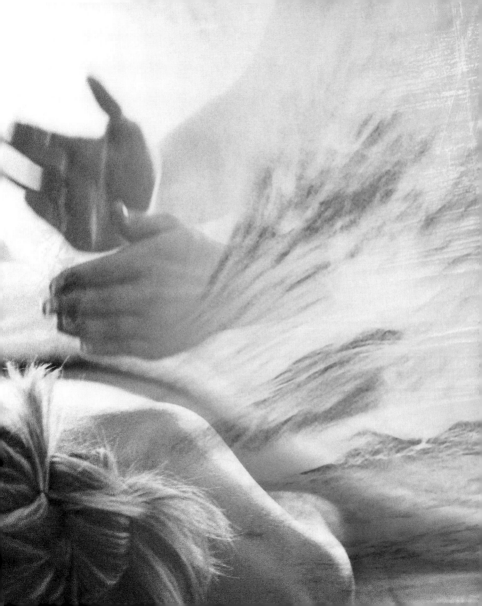

# chapter 2

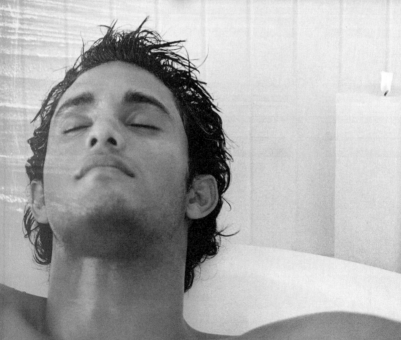

## home **spa** environment

Your home spa environment is a place for you to recharge and revitalise. You therefore want it to be clean and fresh. Let's start with the bathroom because that is where many of your home spa treatments will take place (see Chapter 5 for treatments).

First, clean everything in the bathroom. Discard anything you do not use or haven't used in the past six months, especially any unused beauty products that you want to hang on to for that 'one day' that never comes. Now run your eye over the following checklist of items and ingredients that I recommend you keep in the bathroom to use regularly.

- ✓ Fresh and clean cotton towels and face cloths. (Wash at least weekly.)
- ✓ Candles. Use natural beeswax candles if possible, as they are non-toxic and non-polluting.

✓ Plants – real, not artificial. Plants can thrive in the moist environment of your bathroom. They look good too and infuse the space with natural energy.

✓ Heater if cold. Make sure it's kept in a safe place away from water and fabrics.

✓ Vaporizer.

✓ Premium quality pure essential oils. (See Chapter 4.)

✓ Fragrance free daily body oils and a shallow dish or glass measure.

✓ Dark glass bottles.

Of course, you'll have your usual bathroom items as well, such as toothpaste and toothbrush, and body care products that you love. Everything you use regularly keep at arm's reach. The dark glass bottles you can store in the vanity cupboard. (You use the bottles to store your aromatherapy blends.)

And you thought the bathroom was simply a place you went to wash! Not anymore. It's a place to nurture and comfort yourself, and you can use every moment you spend in the bathroom to your advantage. Even if it's just to wash your hands. The idea is to create a warm and inviting space so that every time you're in it you feel equipped for change.

A vaporizer, plants, candles, even low-wattage lighting, helps create such a space, so before you do anything else make sure your bathroom is prepared.

Then, it's time to prepare your bedroom. Most spa treatments will take place in the bathroom, but it's important that the environment in the bedroom is also conducive to relaxation, because that's where you'll go after you've been to the bathroom – to either dress or sleep.

Your bedroom should be a nurturing space where you feel safe and relaxed. If it's not already, run your eye over the following checklist.

✓ Clean, fresh cotton sheets. (Wash at least weekly.)

✓ Vaporizer (yes, a separate one for the bedroom) and essential oils. (See Chapter 4 for compendium of essential oils.)

✓ Candles. Again, use beeswax candles as they are non-toxic and non-polluting, and they don't emit poisonous fumes. Also, use bedside lamps rather than overhead lights, as they create an environment that is more gentle and relaxed.

✓ A glass bottle fitted with a spray top. Fill the glass bottle with water and add 2 drops of essential oil as it's a great wake-me-up in the morning. Try a rosemary and lemon, or bergamot and grapefruit blend – simply close your eyes and spray on your face as soon as you wake up to help you break from the sleep state and get your day started. You can also use the glass bottle to scent your sheets and pillows with an aromatic mist. Use oils that relax rather than stimulate, such as lavender. (See Chapter 4 for more information.)

✓ Try to make it a habit to strip the bed monthly (everything including the underlay) and spritz the mattress and pillows with a strong aromatic brew. (In a glass bottle with a spray top, add 100mls of purified water and 25 drops of tea tree.) I also spritz the carpet underneath the bed. It's a natural way to clean areas that are prone to dust mites and allergens.

That's a basic list that should contribute to a pleasant bedroom environment that is conducive to romance, rest and relaxation. I also wanted to include a more extensive list based on Feng Shui principles recommended by a very good friend of mine (thanks, Athena). Also known as the Chinese art of placement, Feng Shui aims to create a harmonious environment in and around the home by maximising the chi (energy) in your home.

✓ Remove anything from your bedroom that may disturb your sleep: mirrors, electrical appliances, clutter and too many bright colours. Never sleep with an electric blanket on, as it can disrupt your body's regenerating process. You may wake feeling exhausted or unwell.

✓ Remove any electrical radios or alarm clocks from your bedroom, as your brain is susceptible to electro magnetic energy. It's best to use a battery operated clock in the bedroom, and place it and other appliances as far away from the bed as possible.

✓ Whenever possible, scent your sheets and pillows with an aromatic mist.

✓ Choose bedspreads that have gentle, simple patterns.

✓ Avoid strong contrasting colours, such as purple next to bright yellow. Also, avoid dark ceilings, which are said to create a dead, lifeless energy.

✓ Try to keep anything work-related out of the bedroom. If you do have a computer in the bedroom, cover it at night and place an amethyst crystal next to it.

✓ Try not to store anything under the bed, as it disrupts the flow of chi, and clean under it regularly to shift stagnant energy.

✓ To enhance rest and relaxation, vaporize lavender, marjoram, orange, mandarin and chamomile.

✓ To enhance intimacy and romance, vaporize ylang ylang, patchouli, jasmine, rose and sandalwood.

✓ Take an aromatic bath using essential oils that promote sleep: Lavender, orange, mandarin and marjoram.

By implementing these simple tips, you can transform your bedroom into a private sanctuary where you can nurture and care for yourself.

I'm sure you'll discover many other ways to enhance your home spa environment as you go. Now it's time to find out more about aromatherapy, and how you can use it to create the quintessential home spa experience.

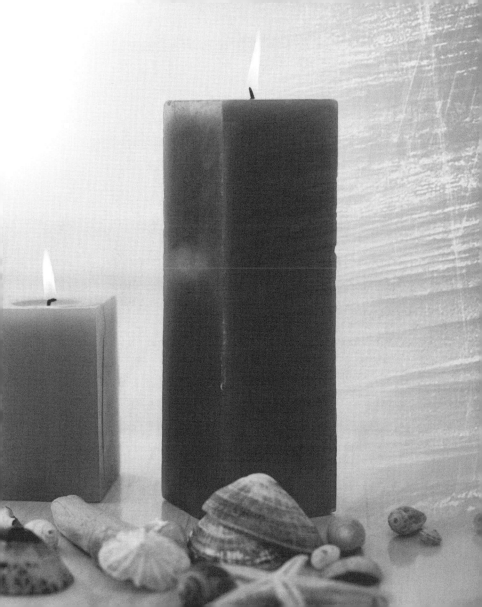

# chapter 3

# home **spa** aromatherapy

My experience of aromatherapy as a practitioner, teacher, author, mother and wife is extensive. I have pooled that knowledge to share with you secrets on how to enhance your home spa treatments. As I mentioned in the introduction, it was my love of essential oils that first inspired the idea for *Home Spa*; that is, how to use it to create a spa environment at home. That's the beauty of aromatherapy; you don't need a practitioner to administer it; with a bit of common-sense and practical know-how, aromatherapy is a modality that is safe to practice in your own home – you only need to follow some simple directions. And when you start to incorporate the use of essential oils into your daily routine, you'll notice an overall improvement in the way you deal with life. Your energy levels will increase and you'll find more time to spend on other things besides physical ailments, mental fatigue and stress.

Whether inhaled, diluted and massaged into the skin, or prepared for a compress, bath or shower, premium quality pure essential oils (preferably organic) go to work to heal and balance the body. However, the word 'oil' is somewhat misleading, because essential oils are not oily like sweet almond oil or macadamia oil; they are volatile liquids that evaporate when exposed to the air. They act quickly when applied, diffusing through your skin and even penetrating the walls of your blood vessels and body tissues. This is why it's important to never compromise on quality when it comes to buying essential oils.

When they are first absorbed, essential oils diffuse and settle in various regions of your body until you begin to metabolise and excrete them through urination, perspiration and respiration. Although they can take up to four hours to diffuse throughout the body, they will not remain in your system for more than a few hours; sufficient time to trigger the body's ability to heal, which can continue for a few days.

Essential oils dissolve readily into body fat (the more body fat you have the more you'll absorb) and then pass to your central nervous system and liver. The brain is very rich in fat, which leads scientists to speculate that it easily takes up fat-soluble molecules such as essential oils and that they remain there for some time, hence the prolonged psychological effects of essential oils on our emotions.

Once the essential oils are absorbed into the body, a whole range of chemical reactions take place. The body takes what it needs from the oils and the remainder is transformed into water-soluble molecules and excreted. The body makes use of the oils to prevent any attack from bacteria, viruses, fungi, parasites, allergens and toxins. So, the simple act of moisturising your skin daily can create a powerful defence against disease.

In contrast to sweating, which is an active, energy-demanding process, diffusion of the oils through the skin occurs quite passively – the skin cells don't pump the essential oil molecules to the deeper layers of the skin, they sink in naturally.

The amount of an essential oil blend that is diffused depends on the colour, quality, function, fat content and size of the surface area of your skin that you rub it into. Ultimately, the more skin you cover with your essential oil blend, the greater the dose. However, it's important to note that some oils can effectively treat conditions in very small amounts.

The skin is the largest organ of the body and can cover – depending on your age, size and shape – approximately 1.8 metres in surface area. It contains metres of blood vessels, thousands of nerve endings, hundreds of sweat glands and millions of cells. It also eliminates waste and manufactures vitamins. And with thousands of sensory nerve endings, it warns you of danger and allows you to enjoy lots of pleasure.

The nose is another way for essential oils to pass into the body. Because they are volatile, they are easily inhaled, and once inhaled they reach the olfactory epithelium, a small patch located at the top of your nasal cavity which contains about five million receptor cells that can recognise about 10,000 different smells. The brain then registers the essential oil – as pleasant, neutral or unpleasant – and sends the information to the rest of the body. After the molecules are recognised by the brain, they pass down the nasal cavity to the trachea and into the bronchii before they complete a journey to the lungs.

Our sense of smell is intrinsically linked to memory, and we record our associations to smells in the limbic centre, the same part of the brain where we process memory. Therefore, a healthy way to use essential oils in your daily life is to link a pleasant essential oil odour to a pleasant association and use it to heal. For example, the smell of jasmine may remind you of a happy time in your childhood. You can then use the smell of jasmine as an adult to recall the happy experience; the smell is registered by the brain and then instigates a rush of 'good' chemicals to the body.

Anecdotal reports also suggest that essential oils – when they penetrate the bloodstream and reach the limbic centre of the brain – can alter the chemistry of the body. The oils have a life-promoting effect, which helps improve the health of your body.

Essential oils are indeed catalysts for change. They can alter the way we think and feel in just a few seconds, and that's why they are such an essential tool for your home spa.

Each essential oil has its own aroma and healing ability. Like fingerprints, each one is unique. Even essential oils from the same botanical family can smell slightly different. Roses grown in Bulgaria smell slightly sweeter than roses grown in France, which often smell more woody. That's because the soils and environmental conditions of the country directly affect the aromatics of plants.

In the same way that no two essential oils are absolutely identical, no two people will experience an essential oil in exactly the same way. It's a personal journey, so it's up to you which oils you decide to use.

You may choose an oil for its fragrance, or for its physical effects on the body. Or you might choose an oil because it lifts your spirits and balances your emotions.

Essential oils are *the* most important items in *Home Spa*, and it's helpful to understand how they interact with the body. As I've already mentioned, essential oils can not only have a physical effect on the body, they can also affect the way we feel and think. Though we can't yet measure the effects, anyone who has ever smelled a wild rose knows that the beauty of the scent and the majesty of the bloom have a magnetic power over the mind and the emotions. That's the beauty of smell.

And now with the theory out of the way, let's get practical.

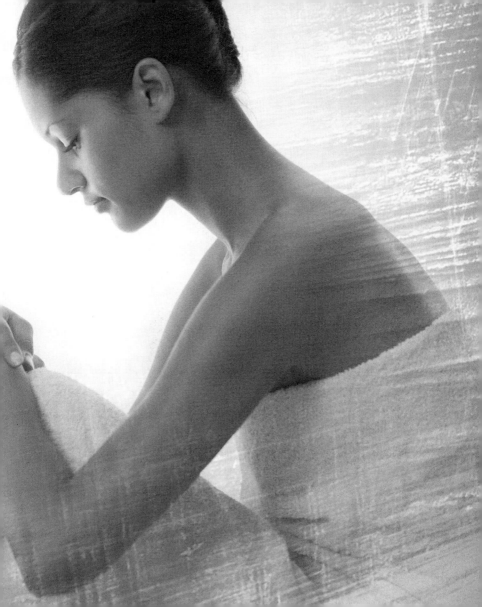

chapter 4

## a **compendium** of **26 essential** oils

In *home spa*, essential oils are your main ingredient, and the more you know about each oil, the greater its use. The following 26 oils make up the essential oil range I formulated, called Cross-Cultural Essential Oils (please see: Organic and Cross-Cultural Essential Oils' at back of book). You can choose to use my organic aromatherapy range or any other high quality range. Remember, essential oil molecules pass through the skin's epidermis and are absorbed by the capillary blood that circulates in the dermis of the skin, so you want to make sure they are of high quality. It's important to never compromise on quality because when you do you compromise on health.

To ensure you choose a quality brand, I suggest you carefully read the guidelines on the label. Quality essential oils should carry warnings, such as:

✓ for external use only.

✓ keep out of reach of children.

✓ if ingested by a child, seek urgent medical help.

✓ essential oils can irritate if used undiluted.

✓ never use near the eyes or on diseased or damaged skin, unless advised by an authorised practitioner.

✓ never use them on the skin (massage) during the first three months of pregnancy.

Some additional precautions (less likely to appear on the packaging yet important all the same) include:

✓ when added to water, always agitate the surface to disperse the essential oil molecules.

✓ when breastfeeding halve the recommended adult dosage when applying topically and avoid the breast and nipple area.

✓ avoid topical application of essential oils on infants less than two years of age. For specific infant treatments, say, diaper rash, always halve the dosage recommended for children.

✓ do not apply essential oils near or on the eye or genital areas.

✓ if skin irritation occurs due to the use of an aromatherapy, blend, dilute or remove it with a cold-pressed oil, not water.

✓ prolonged inhalation of essential oils (sniffing directly from bottle) should be avoided as it could cause lightheadedness, headaches, vertigo, nausea or lethargy.

✓ if essential oils are ingested (especially by a child), seek immediate professional advice.

✓ avoid citrus oils on the skin for up to 12 hours prior to sunbathing or exposure to UV light.

✓ do not use essential oils undiluted on the skin. Unless directed otherwise, dilute essential oils in a fragrance-free body oil such as sweet almond, peach kernel, macadamia nut, jojoba, evening primrose or rosehip before application to the skin. (One drop of tea tree oil added to the end of a cotton bud and dabbed directly onto a pimple is an exception to the rule.)

✓ pregnant women should always halve the recommended adult dosage for any topical application of essential oils that are listed as safe to use after the first trimester (see page 92 – Massage and Pregnancy). Avoid topical application of the following essential oils during pregnancy: Basil, clary sage, cedarwood, cypress, eucalyptus, lemongrass, lime, fennel, frankincense, ginger, marjoram, peppermint, rosemary, rose, sage, tea tree and thyme.

As a final precautionary note, even if the oils you use are thought to be completely safe, natural and pure, there is always a slim chance of a one in a million idiosyncratic response. Some people simply react adversely to an otherwise completely safe substance or material. If this happens to you, treat it in the same way you would any other adverse physiological reaction and seek prompt medical attention. You can always help remove essential oils by diluting them on the skin with a cold-pressed oil (such as olive oil) or fat (such as butter). If you accidentally wipe essential oils into the delicate eye area, then bathe the eye with cold milk.

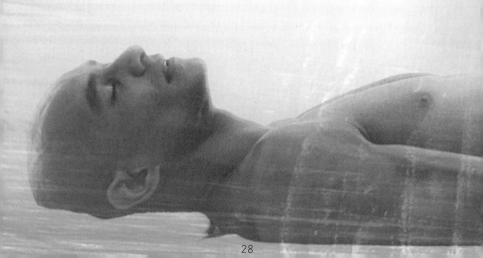

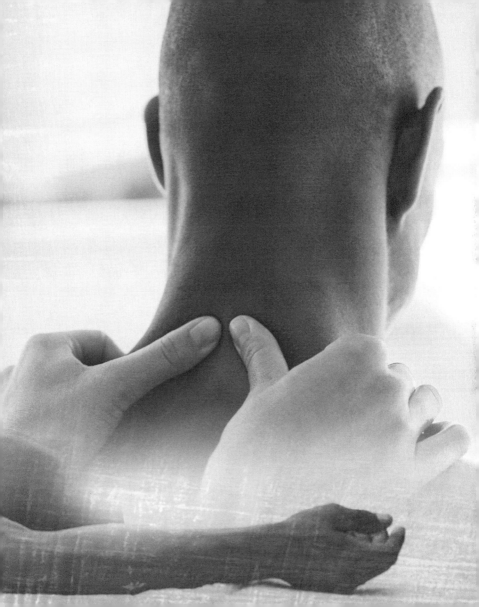

# Basil

= **key** words: Enthusiasm, clarification and focus

= **botanical** name: *Ocimum basilicum* (be sure to use the linalool chemo type with low estragole content between 1.3 and 16.5%)

= **countries** of origin: Egypt, India and France

= **derived** from: The herb flower

= **blends well** with: Bergamot, cedarwood, clary sage, eucalyptus, frankincense, geranium, grapefruit, jasmine, lavender, lemon, lemongrass, lime, mandarin, marjoram, neroli, orange, patchouli, rosemary and rosewood

= virtues: Basil treats apprehension, confusion, nervous exhaustion, lethargy, depression, loss of memory, irregular periods, spasmodic coughing, headaches and migraines, indigestion and wasp stings; it is used in the treatment of herpes and shingles and also acts as a mosquito repellent

= skin care: Improves sluggish and congested skin (use sparingly); stimulates hair growth and improves hair lustre

= precautions: Avoid the basil estragole chemo type (it has a high methyl chavicol – estragole – content of 40 to 87%, which can be carcinogenic); avoid topical application during pregnancy; avoid on sensitive and damaged skin; do not take orally; keep out of reach of children; follow directions for use and dosage recommendations

= Basil encourages enthusiasm. If you feel confused, basil helps settle the mind as it has a clarifying effect on the brain. Its aroma can sharpen your intuition and assist you when you need to make important decisions. It is also extremely effective for relieving mental fatigue.

Physically, basil is an appetite stimulant and digestive aid. It is also excellent as a chest rub for respiratory ailments such as bronchitis, coughs and colds, and is a fantastic nerve tonic, inspiring strength and energy. Emotionally, it can be used to activate your 'appetite for life'. Purpose and focus are the attributes inspired by the oil.

Basil is an ideal choice if you're just about to conduct or attend a business conference, or for any environment where you wish to encourage focused participation as it helps people concentrate on important data.

# Bergamot

= **key** words: Spontaneity, versatility and encouragement

= **botanical** name: *Citrus bergamia*

= **countries** of origin: Italy, Sicily and Ivory Coast

= **derived** from: The peel of the fruit

= **blends well** with: Basil, Roman chamomile, cedarwood, clary sage, eucalyptus, frankincense, geranium, grapefruit, lavender, lemon, lemongrass, lime, mandarin, neroli, orange, patchouli, rose, rosemary, sandalwood, tea tree and ylang ylang

= **virtues:** Stimulates appetite and relieves nervousness; counteracts stress, nervous anxiety, melancholy and depression; treats skin disorders such as eczema, dermatitis and acne; assists the healing of wounds and sores; helps treat intestinal parasites, adult colic, urinary infections and cramps; supports general wellbeing

= **skin care:** Assists healing (especially eczema and dermatitis) as it's highly antiseptic; helps treat acne, boils, cold sores and seborrhoea of skin and scalp; insect repellent

= precautions: Bergamot is phototoxic, which means it shouldn't be used externally before exposure to ultra-violet light for up to 12 hours following application; may irritate highly sensitive skin; avoid topical application during the first three months of pregnancy; do not take orally; keep out of reach of children; follow directions for use and dosage recommendations

= Bergamot inspires spontaneity and light heartedness, and is pure delight for the senses. It has a cooling effect which quells anxiety, promoting general wellbeing and the flow of energy throughout the body. When things seem 'stuck', bergamot can bring movement and flow. Its antiseptic nature has a refreshing quality, which is great for relieving the symptoms associated with melancholy and depression. It encourages you to 'let go'.

Inhale a few drops of bergamot whenever you feel nervous, as it helps release pent up emotions and concerns. It's great if you are a teacher, presenter or facilitator, as it can help calm pre-presentation jitters.

# Cedarwood

- = **key** words: Certainty, stability and inner strength
- = **botanical** name: *Cedrus atlantica*
- = **countries** of origin: North Africa and Morocco
- = **derived** from: The wood
- = **blends well** with: Basil, bergamot, eucalyptus, frankincense, geranium, grapefruit, jasmine, lavender, lemon, lemongrass, lime, mandarin, marjoram, neroli, orange, rosewood, sandalwood and ylang ylang
- = virtues: Helps to regulate the nervous system, nervous debility, emotional instability, mental strain, chronic anxiety, tension, fear, anger and disconnectedness; kills air-borne bacteria; helps flaky skin conditions such as dermatitis, eczema, dandruff, psoriasis, seborrhoea of the scalp and acne; treats chest conditions such as catarrh and bronchial coughs; addresses genito-urinary infections including vaginitis and cystitis
- = skin care: The anti-ageing quality of this oil helps to improve the quality of oily skin and prevents acne; addresses fungal infections, chronic dermatitis and sites that ooze pus; helps dandruff and alopecia; reduces the appearance of cellulite

= precautions: Avoid topical application during pregnancy; do not take orally; keep out of reach of children; follow directions for use and dosage recommendations

= Cedarwood is relaxing and is said to inspire certainty and reassurance. It helps steady and ground the mind, and so provides the strength to be steadfast during times of trauma or crisis. A great oil when life demands a lot.

Cedarwood can assist chest complaints such as catarrh and bronchitis, and can decongest and strengthen the lungs. It also helps cleanse the body and can assist weight loss. Used in conjunction with rosemary, it can help to restore hair growth.

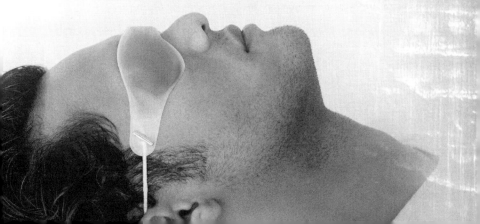

# Chamomile [Roman]

= **key** words: Patience, serenity and tenderness

= **botanical** name: *Anthemis nobilis*

= **countries** of origin: Switzerland, Hungary, USA, France and Italy

= **derived** from: The flowers

= **blends well** with: Bergamot, clary sage, geranium, jasmine, lavender, mandarin, marjoram, neroli, rose, rosewood and sandalwood

= **virtues**: Assists conditions such as nervous tension, hypersensitivity, unstable emotions, irritability, anger and fear, PMS, rheumatism, gout, flatulence, dermatitis and conjunctivitis; effective treatment for irritated skin as well as irritable bowel, gastric and menstrual discomfort; helps treat anaemia, loss of appetite and allergic reactions

= **skin care**: Relieves and soothes red and blotchy skin, allergic reactions and boils; soothes dry, itchy, irritated and hypersensitive skin; reduces puffiness and darkness under eye area (use with extreme caution: Dilute oil and apply compress to outer eye socket only, rest with eyes closed for 10 minutes and remove)

= precautions: Avoid topical application during the first three months of pregnancy; do not take orally; keep out of reach of children; follow directions for use and dosage recommendations

= Chamomile is renowned for its ability to arouse sleep, yet that is the least of its benefits. Chamomile has remarkable anti-inflammatory and anti-bacterial powers. It is also purifying, soothing and calming, and has the ability to increase the production of white corpuscles, which aid healing and boost the immune system.

When used in conjunction with massage, it can effectively treat gout and rheumatism. It has been used for centuries to treat neuralgia, menopausal symptoms, and gastric and intestinal problems. It helps to soothe and regenerate wounds, herpes, eczema and other skin irritations.

# Clary Sage

= **key** words: Euphoric, reviving and exciting

= **botanical** name: *Salvia sclarea*

= **countries** of origin: France, Russia, China and USA

= **derived** from: The flowers

= **blends well** with: Basil, bergamot, Roman chamomile, geranium, grapefruit, jasmine, lavender, mandarin, neroli, patchouli, rose, sandalwood and ylang ylang

= virtues: Brings clarity when in a transitional phase of life; helps counteract depression, postnatal depression, over-sensitivity, uncontrollable emotions, paranoia, nightmares and despondency; helps to regulate menstruation and reduces abdominal cramps, PMS, menopausal hot flushes and frigidity; relieves tired and aching legs; good for oily skin and hair; reduces appearance of cellulite

= skin care: Cell regenerator, especially for ageing skin; treats acne and boils; helps regulate production of sebum to prevent dandruff

= precautions: Avoid topical application during pregnancy; do not take orally; keep out of reach of children; follow directions for use and dosage recommendations

= This is the most euphoric of all the essential oils. It is a particularly effective treatment for stress-related problems. It is also a wonderful revival tonic, good for the treatment of fatigue.

The Latin botanical name for clary sage translates as 'clear', and it is renowned for its ability to restore clarity as it dispels nervous anxiety and confusion. Insight and intuition become more acute when clary sage is used.

Clary sage helps young people ease into adolescence when emotional and physical changes are dramatic. It is also useful during menopause, as it supports the sensitive transition from mid-life to later life.

# Eucalyptus

= **key** words: Antiseptic, invigorating and clearing

= **botanical** name: *Eucalyptus globulus*

= **countries** of origin: China, Australia and Paraguay

= **derived** from: The leaves

= **blends well** with: Basil, bergamot, cedarwood, frankincense, grapefruit, lemon, lemongrass, lime, peppermint, rosemary and tea tree

= **virtues:** Good for melancholic moods, exhaustion, lack of concentration and irrational behaviour; helps treat respiratory disorders, coughs, colds, flu, sinusitis, bronchitis, catarrh and viral conditions; helps clear infection; relieves muscular aches and

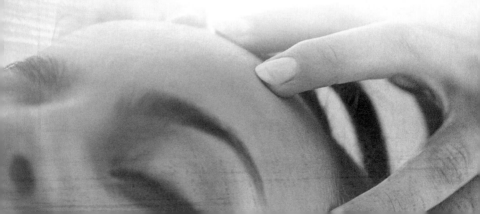

pains; helps reduce high temperatures and fevers associated with measles and infection; relieves rheumatism and arthritis

= skin care: Decongests sluggish skin (especially for cigarette smokers); treats burns, blisters, cuts and insect bites; treats lice; reduces skin and bacterial infections; improves circulation

= precautions: Avoid topical application during pregnancy; avoid use if you have high blood pressure or epilepsy; do not store with homeopathic remedies; do not take orally; keep out of reach of children; follow directions for use and dosage

= When you need encouragement, use eucalyptus, as it helps promote a positive outlook. Its energising and stimulating qualities can bring a new perspective to any situation.

Inhale eucalyptus to clear the head and inspire rational thought. With its refreshing and invigorating qualities, eucalyptus can help you get motivated.

Eucalyptus is one of the most powerful antiviral essential oils and is wonderful for coughs, colds and flu; it is also a decongestant that can clear the sinuses. It is a great immune system booster as well as a general body tonic, as it promotes oxygen uptake in the body.

# Frankincense

= **key** words: Tranquillity, spirituality and security

= **botanical** name: *Boswellia carterii*

= **countries** of origin: Oman, Arabia and Somalia

= **derived** from: The gum of the tree

= **blends well** with: Basil, bergamot, cedarwood, eucalyptus, grapefruit, jasmine, lavender, lemon, lemongrass, lime, marjoram, peppermint, rose, rosemary, sandalwood and tea tree

= virtues: Ideal for healing; helps treat old emotional wounds, emotional or mental anguish, depression, paranoia, nightmares and irrational fears; good for weeping sores, wounds, aggravated joints (rheumatism), ulcerated skin, stress-related conditions and post-operative scars; can be useful in the treatment of diarrhoea, chronic burping, fluid retention and bronchial irritation; useful in weight loss programs

= skin care: Helps rejuvenate dry, mature skin and smooth out wrinkles; good for oily skin; helps repair and heal the superficial layers of the skin; relieves acne, pimples, scars and ulcers

= precautions: Avoid topical application during pregnancy; do not take orally; keep out of reach of children; follow directions for use and dosage recommendations

= Frankincense instils tranquillity. It can also enhance blissful states in meditation, and is renowned for its use throughout history to dismiss negative energy in spiritual and religious rites. It was often used as an incense to expand consciousness and awaken the spirit. It's also helpful when you need to make important life decisions.

Frankincense is a mild diuretic and can help to dispel irrational fears, paranoia and nightmares. Inhaled, it can help to comfort even the most nervous individuals. Blends well with cedarwood to relieve catarrhal conditions.

Frankincense can also be used as a skin tonic, especially for mature skin, to revitalise and regenerate.

# Geranium

- = **key** words: Balance, composure and sensitivity
- = **botanical** name: *Pelaragonium graveolens*
- = **countries** of origin: Egypt, China and Morocco
- = **derived** from: The herb
- = **blends well** with: Basil, bergamot, Roman chamomile, cedar-wood, clary sage, jasmine, lavendar, lemongrass, mandarin, marjoram, neroli, orange, patchouli, rose, rosewood and sandalwood
- = **virtues**: Helps balance and settle the mind, body and emotions and so assist when you are feeling overwhelmed, are experiencing mood swings or when more flexibility is needed; helps relieve nervous tension, anxiety, PMS, some of the symptoms of menopause and an irregular menstrual cycle; helpful in the treatment of eczema, shingles and chaffedor bruised skin; relieves neuralgia, rheumatism and lymphatic congestion
- = **skin care**: Promotes healing; normalises sebum production; antiseptic and astringent; relieves ulcers, acne, bruises, broken capillaries, congested and mature skin; aids healing after facial surgery when blended with lavender; acts as mosquito repellent

= precautions: Do not use topically on inflamed or damaged skin; avoid topical application during the first three months of pregnancy; do not take orally; keep out of reach of children; follow directions for use and dosage recommendations

= Geranium helps balance the emotional highs and lows of life to bring a sense of calm and assuredness. When you inhale geranium, you may instantly feel more stable and at ease. During times of rapid change and uncertainty, it can help you regain emotional composure and so respond to change with sensitivity and equilibrium.

On a physical and emotional level, it is an excellent choice for postnatal women. It also helps the body to balance dramatic hormonal changes during menopause and puberty.

# Grapefruit

= **key** words: Alert, confident and active

= **botanical** name: *Citrus X paradisi*

= **countries** of origin: Israel, USA and Australia

= **derived** from: The peel of the fruit

= **blends well** with: Basil, bergamot, cedarwood, clary sage, euca-lyptus, frankincense, jasmine, lemon, lemongrass, lime, neroli, orange, patchouli, rosemary and tea tree

= **virtues**: Counteracts lethargy, negative thinking, despondency, dependency, depression, anxiety and self-doubt; used in the treatment of anorexia or bulimia; stimulates a sluggish lymphatic system and improves peripheral circulation; helps reduce muscle fatigue; blended with clary sage it assists with alcohol and drug withdrawal; reduces the appearance of cellulite

= **skin care**: Promotes circulation; cleanses the skin; relieves Athlete's foot, acne and oily skin; when blended with lemon and clary sage it helps tighten and tone the skin; use with rose-mary to stimulate hair growth

= precautions: Grapefruit may be photosensitive, therefore avoid topical application for up to 12 hours before exposure to ultraviolet light; avoid topical application during the first three months of pregnancy; do not take orally; keep out of reach of children; follow directions for use and dosage recommendations

= Grapefruit sharpens the senses and boosts confidence and reassurance. Use it to promote spontaneity and light heartedness, especially when feeling overwhelmed or depressed.

Use grapefruit during any weight loss program because it helps settle anxiety and provide comfort when food cravings occur. It activates liver function and promotes the production of bile, and is therefore a great digestive aid. It also has mild diuretic properties and can assist in the breakdown of fats in the body. Good for cellulite treatments.

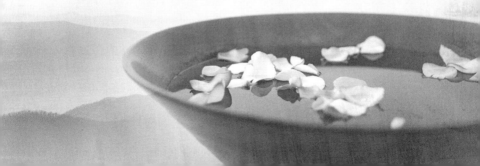

# Jasmine Absolute

= **key** words: Intoxicating, enchanting and sensual

= **botanical** name: *Jasminum grandiflorum*

= **countries** of origin: France and Egypt

= **derived** from: The flower

= **blends well** with: Basil, Roman chamomile, cedarwood, clary sage, frankincense, geranium, grapefruit, lavender, marjoram, orange, patchouli, rose, rosewood, sandalwood, ylang ylang

= **virtues**: Helps dispel irrational fears, nervous anxiety, vulnerability, pessimism, low self-esteem, guilt, frigidity, impotence, labour pains, PMS, menopausal symptoms, painful periods; eases muscular aches and pains including abdominal cramps; when blended with lavender, treats headaches and helps protect against bacterial infections, dermatitis and catarrhal conditions

= **skin care**: Softens and soothes dry, irritated skin; ideal for mature skin or skin that is ageing prematurely; can be used to help repair stretch marks

= precautions: Avoid topical application during the first three months of pregnancy and on sensitive and broken skin; do not take orally; keep out of reach of children; follow directions for use and dosage recommendations

= Emotionally, jasmine can inspire you to feel more optimistic. Physically, it helps to regulate the female reproductive system and relieve PMS and period pain. Warm and seductive, jasmine oil has also been used as an aphrodisiac for many thousands of years.

Jasmine is beneficial for dry and mature skin, stretch marks, joint pains and dermatitis. On a more subtle level, jasmine is said to stimulate the creative urge; artists are inspired to paint, sing, dance, sculpt and write in the presence of this fragrance.

# Lavender

- = **key** words: Soothing, nurturing and calming
- = **botanical** name: *Lavandula angustifolia*
- = **countries** of origin: Bulgaria, France, Australia, England, Mongolia and Ukraine
- = **derived** from: The flowering tops
- = **blends well** with: Basil, bergamot, Roman chamomile, cedarwood, clary sage, frankincense, geranium, jasmine, mandarin, marjoram, neroli, orange, patchouli, rose, rosewood, sandalwood, tea tree and ylang ylang
- = virtues: Ideal for impatience, irritability, mood swings, anger, hysteria, over-sensitivity; helps anxiety and stress; antiviral and antibacterial; good for skin repair: scar tissue, eczema, psoriasis, dermatitis, mosquito and insect bites
- = skin care: Rejuvenates cells and helps heal; treats eczema, psoriasis, burns, bruises and scars; soothes any irritation or injury; helps treat acne, and dry, oily and combination skin

= precautions: Avoid topical application during the first three months of pregnancy; do not take orally; keep out of reach of children; follow directions for use and dosage recommendations

= Lavender helps soothe the heart and allay nervous anxiety and panic. Use it to counteract trauma or during a difficult time, as it helps release restrained emotions and restores equilibrium.

Lavender has many actions: It works as an anti-bacterial agent, stimulates cell growth and works as a gentle sedative. At night, an active or restless child can often be calmed with just a single drop on a pillow.

With powerful anti-inflammatory actions it can cool and treat any type of burn, skin inflammation and/or infection, including insect bites and stings. An ideal post-operative treatment.

The analgesic properties of lavender help reduce the pain of headaches and migraines, and settle sensations of dizziness often associated with these conditions. An excellent general tonic, it is useful during convalescence, as it nurtures, heals and strengthens.

# Lemon

- = **key** words: Lively, perceptive and clear
- = **botanical** name: *Citrus limonum*
- = **countries** of origin: Spain, Italy, Israel, USA, Australia and Argentina
- = **derived** from: Peel of the fruit
- = **blends well** with: Basil, bergamot, cedarwood, eucalyptus, frankincense, grapefruit, lime, neroli, orange, peppermint, rosemary and tea tree
- = virtues: Assists irritability, indecision, lethargy and tiredness; helps reduce liver congestion, flatulence (intestinal gas), gall stones, kidney stones; addresses respiratory disorders such as colds, flu and bronchitis; strengthens broken capillaries, weak nails and hair; treats oily skin, warts and fluid retention
- = skin care: Cleanses; treats acne, boils, corns and warts; strengthens connective tissue; excellent as a toner or astringent for oily skin; improves circulation
- = precautions: Lemon is phototoxic, therefore avoid topical application for up to 12 hours before exposure to ultraviolet light; avoid

topical application during the first three months of pregnancy and on sensitive skin; do not take orally; keep out of reach of children; follow directions for use and dosage recommendations

= The light, clear, refreshing fragrance of lemon uplifts the spirit and cleanses the mind. If in doubt or confused, lemon brings focus and clarity. A mind weighed down with uncertainty can be uplifted and positively energised with the zest of lemon.

Lemon also boosts concentration, alertness and productivity. A blend of lemon, basil and rosemary can help focus the mind and deliver results. Research carried out by the Shimizu Corporation in Japan showed that vaporizing lemon in the workplace helped to increase productivity and decrease work error by a minimum of 35%.

Lemon oil helps the body defend itself against infections, especially respiratory conditions when catarrh is present. It is also an excellent cleanser and effective if you need to combat airborne viruses and bacteria. Blended with eucalyptus and tea tree, lemon is ideal if you want to detoxify your system. It also works as a natural disinfectant.

It is useful in the treatment of oily and congested skin, and aids circulation.

# Lemongrass

= **key** words: Revitalizing, activating and releasing

= **botanical** name: *Cymbopogon flexuosus*

= **countries** of origin: India, Guatemala and Sri Lanka

= **derived** from: The herb grass

= **blends well** with: Basil, bergamot, cedarwood, eucalyptus, frankincense, geranium, grapefruit, lime, neroli, rosemary and sandalwood

= virtues: Useful for stress-related conditions; relieves chronic anxiety; reduces the appearance of cellulite; immune stimulant; tonifying for the skin and muscles; treats oily, congested and acne skin; works as an astringent

= skin care: Stimulates lymphatic system; tones the skin; reduces blackheads; cleanses; strengthens connective tissue; reduces appearance of cellulite; detoxifies and deodorizes (reduces foot odour)

= precautions: Avoid topically on sensitive or damaged skin; avoid topical application during pregnancy and on babies and children (oil for adult use only); do not take orally; keep out of reach of children; follow directions for use and dosage recommendations

= Lemongrass has been used in purification rituals, and in Asian, Mexican and South American cooking for eons. It encourages flexibility and movement, even in the most fixed personality.

It is fortifying to the nervous system, especially for those who persevere in spite of feeling vulnerable and overwhelmed. Lemongrass disperses underlying tension and anxiety, and helps to tone and cleanse the whole body. As a powerful tonic, it has the capacity to revive and revitalise a weary body. It also acts as an immune stimulant. Its ability to stimulate and activate has been known to reduce lactic acid after physical activity, as well as tone muscles and connective tissue. It's therefore good to use for weight loss and post-exercise recovery. With its anti-microbial properties, it can act as a potent antiseptic and is great as a disinfectant. It is also indicated to treat bacterial infections.

# Lime

- = **key** words: Assertive, attentive and energetic
- = **botanical** name: *Citrus aurantifolia*
- = **countries** of origin: Peru, Mexico, Ivory Coast and USA
- = **derived** from: The peel of the fruit
- = **blends well** with: Basil, bergamot, cedarwood, eucalyptus, frankincense, grapefruit, lemon, lemongrass, neroli, peppermint, rosemary and tea tree
- = virtues: Helps with melancholy, apathy, anxiety, negativity; restores self worth; improves concentration; refreshes a tired mind and can be used for the treatment of dementia; reduces severity of chest and respiratory conditions such as asthma, bronchitis, congestion, flu and sore throat; may assist muscle spasms, cramps, lymphatic congestion, fluid retention, flatulence and obesity
- = skin care: Effective deodorant that helps cleanse and purify; eases inflammation, although avoid on sensitive and damaged skin; acts as an astringent to tighten and tone the skin

= precautions: Lime is photosensitive, therefore avoid topical application for up to 12 hours before exposure to ultraviolet light; avoid application to damaged and sensitive skin, dermal irritant; avoid topical application during the first three months of pregnancy; do not take orally; keep out of reach of children; follow directions for use and dosage recommendations

= Lime oil has refreshing qualities that uplift and revitalise the nervous system. It can inspire a positive outlook and dispel apathy, and is especially good for those who feel melancholy or listless. Lime is also good for assertiveness, especially when hopes are high but spirits are low. Use lime as a great pick-me-up for exhaustion.

Lime is also an excellent oil for elderly people who have a problem with memory recall. It helps activate the mind and engage the intellect.

With antibacterial properties, lime also helps cleanse the body. It is an excellent addition to any weight loss program as it can help reduce fluid retention. As an antiviral oil, it also benefits the immune system during winter.

# Mandarin

- = **key** words: Happiness, celebration and serenity
- = **botanical** name: *Citrus reticulata*
- = **countries** of origin: Italy, Australia and Sicily
- = **derived** from: The peel of the fruit
- = **blends well** with: Basil, bergamot, Roman chamomile, cedarwood, clary sage, geranium, lavender, marjoram, neroli, orange, patchouli, rosewood, sandalwood and ylang ylang
- = virtues: Good for amnesia, shock and hysteria, grief, depression; helps prevent muscular spasms, constipation, abdominal cramps and PMS, hiccups, stretch marks, congested and oily skin
- = skin care: Treats acne, scars, congested and combination skin; effective skin toner and tonic – moisturises and softens as it strengthens skin; reduces the appearance of stretch marks
- = precautions: Mandarin is photosensitive, therefore avoid topical application for up to 12 hours before exposure to ultraviolet light; avoid topical application during the first three months of pregnancy; do not take orally; keep out of reach of children; follow directions for use and dosage recommendations

= As a remedy for restlessness and uncertainty, mandarin helps soothe worry and tension and bring joy and lightheartedness. A sweet oil, mandarin can inspire an attitude of genuine care and childlike innocence. Therefore, it's of great benefit to people with compulsive behaviours or addictions.

Mandarin also helps bring a restful and deep sleep, especially when combined with lavender and marjoram. It is also an excellent digestive aid, and when massaged onto the abdominal area in a clockwise direction helps relieve intestinal discomfort. Good for meditation, too.

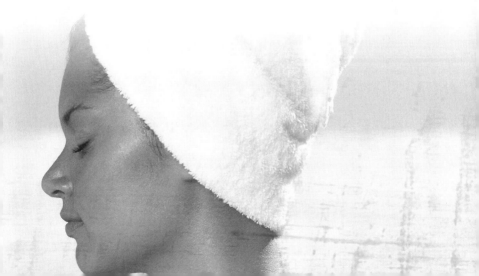

# Marjoram

= **key** words: Deep relaxation, comfort and contentment

= **botanical** name: *Origanum marjorana*

= **countries** of origin: Egypt and France

= **derived** from: The herb

= **blends well** with: Basil, Roman chamomile, cedarwood, frankincense, geranium, grapefruit, jasmine, lavender, mandarin, neroli, orange, rose, rosewood, sandalwood

= **virtues**: Can assist with grief, hostility, anger, hyper-anxiety, emotional extremes, apprehension, nervous tension; treats muscle stiffness, palpitations, cramps and spasms; helps reduce the symptoms associated with bronchitis, asthma, coughs and chronic coughing; aids long-term insomnia and high blood pressure; moderates excessive sexual desire

= **skin care**: Soothes and nourishes the skin; treats chilblains; aids healing of bruises and wounds

= **precautions**: Avoid topical application during pregnancy and with low blood pressure; do not use during deep depression; can cause drowsiness; do not take orally; keep out of reach of children; follow directions for use and dosage recommendations

= In ancient Greece, marjoram was known as a funeral herb, used to ease the journey of the departed spirit. When combined with rose, it is very effective during times of bereavement. Its sedating qualities also promote a deep and restful sleep.

Due to its analgesic and antispasmodic properties, marjoram is excellent for injured and strained muscles. It is a vasodilator and may be a helpful treatment for asthma. It helps relax and relieve tension and pent-up stress in the body. It blends well with lavender and when added to a warm bath before bed (with lavender) can promote deep and restful slumber.

# Neroli

= **key** words: Fulfillment, reassurance and humility

= **botanical** name: *Citrus aurantium var. amara*

= **countries** of origin: Egypt, Iran and Tunisia

= **derived** from: The flower

= **blends well** with: Basil, bergamot, Roman chamomile, cedarwood, clary sage, geranium, grapefruit, jasmine, lavender, lemon, lemongrass, lime, mandarin, marjoram, orange, patchouli, rose, sandalwood and ylang ylang

= virtues: Inspires poise and discernment; helps with depression, emotional frigidity, anxiety, hysteria, apprehension, nerves, insomnia, exhaustion; relieves nervous tension from overwork as well as muscular cramps and spasms, especially in the intestinal tract; reduces symptoms of hormonal imbalance including menopause and PMS; assists with palpitations, inflamed, dry sensitive skin, including broken capillaries.

= skin care: Vein tonic; strengthens capillaries; regenerates cells; soothes; helps treat scars, stretch marks, dry and dull skin, sensitive acne conditions; improves elasticity

= precautions: Avoid topical application during the first three months of pregnancy; can be photosensitive, therefore avoid topical application for up to 12 hours before exposure to ultraviolet light; do not take orally; keep out of reach of children; follow directions for use and dosage recommendations

= Neroli can lift your spirits. It has a calming effect on the cardiovascular system and can reduce palpitations and anxiety attacks. It also has a rejuvenating effect on the skin, improving elasticity, and helps to diminish scars, stretch marks and broken veins.

An immune stimulant, Neroli has the capacity to bring even the most stressed executive to a quiet state of mind. It relieves grief and can prove to be a strong tranquilliser.

Neroli is made from the flowers of the bitter orange tree. The flowers symbolise innocence and love in many folkloric traditions and are often used in European wedding rituals. It takes its name from a 16th century Italian princess, Nerola, who used the flowers to perfume her bathwater and clothes.

# Orange

= **key** words: Exuberance, enthusiasm and creativity

= **botanical** name: *Citrus sinensis*

= **countries** of origin: Australia, Brazil, China, Israel and USA

= **derived** from: The peel of the fruit

= **blends well** with: Basil, bergamot, cedarwood, geranium, grapefruit, jasmine, lavender, lemon, mandarin, marjoram, neroli, pathouli, rosewood, sandalwood and ylang ylang

= **virtues**: Ideal for uneasiness, worry, negativity, pessimism, inflexibility, depression, nervous anxiety, constipation and abdominal cramps associated with poor digestion; helps reduce flatulence and irritable bowel conditions; treats muscular spasms

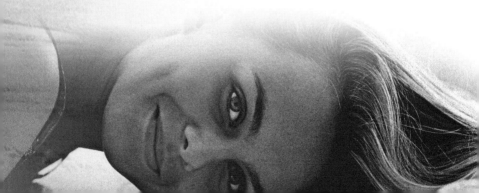

= skin care: Strengthens a weak epidermis and open pores; hydrates the skin; softens hard or cracked skin; good for smoker's skin and cellulite; reduces puffiness; improves circulation

= precautions: Can be photosensitive, so avoid topical application up to 12 hours before exposure to ultraviolet light; avoid on damaged or sensitive skin; avoid topical application first three months of pregnancy; don't use orally; keep out of children's reach; follow directions for use and dosages

= Orange has an energetic, refreshing fragrance which promotes joyful communication. It helps you be more open to new ideas and perspectives, especially if you work in a creative environment.

Orange inspires harmony and therefore helps build co-operation and promotes compatibility. Used daily, it promotes a more positive approach to difficult and confronting tasks. It is excellent when used in meetings to move the conversation forward, and for brainstorming. Also helps to relieve acute headaches or mild insomnia.

Can help to cleanse oily skin, and with its gentle qualities is said to reduce tobacco cravings. Use orange to broaden your imagination and enhance creative visualisation.

# Patchouli

- = **key** words: Exotic, expressive and romantic
- = **botanical** name: *Pogostemon cablin*
- = **countries** of origin: Indonesia, China and Malaysia
- = **derived** from: The leaf
- = **blends well** with: Basil, bergamot, clary sage, geranium, grape-fruit, jasmine, lavender, lime, neroli, orange, rose, rosewood, sandalwood and ylang ylang
- = **virtues**: Assists with apathy, frigidity, impotence, indifference, emotional suppression, depression, anxiety; helps heal open wounds, psoriasis, eczema, acne, dry skin, Athlete's foot, dandruff, scars; reduces the severity of diarrhoea, colon disorders and haemorrhoids; treats fungal infections; eases menopausal sweats
- = **skin care**: Regulates oil secretion and helps reduce open pores; treats fluid retention; can be used to tone slack skin; good for scar tissue, sores, tinea and dry skin
- = **precautions**: May curb appetite; avoid topical application during the first three months of pregnancy; do not take orally; keep

out of reach of children; follow directions for use and dosage recommendations

= Patchouli has a rich aroma and is renowned for its provocative scent; in ancient India it was used as an aphrodisiac. In the 1960s it was used as a perfume to expand consciousness and evoke freedom of sexual expression. It also provides relief from lethargy and anxiety, and can uplift despondent moods.

It works well as an antiseptic to heal cracked, chaffed, loose or broken skin and fungal infections, including Athlete's foot. In old herbal texts from the East, it was said to be of great benefit as an immune stimulant. Old scar tissue responds well to a blend of patchouli and lavender.

# Peppermint

= **key** words: Activating, energizing and clearing

= **botanical** name: *Mentha X. piperita*

= **countries** of origin: USA, England, France and Australia

= **derived** from: The leaf

= **blends well** with: Eucalyptus, frankincense, lemon, lime, rosemary and tea tree

= virtues: Ideal for fatigue, lethargy and lack of focus; relieves the symptoms associated with indigestion, travel sickness, nausea, menstrual cramps and nerve pain

= skin care: Cooling affect on the skin; decongestant (blends well with eucalyptus and tea tree), especially good for acne; relieves itching; treats blackheads; helps rehydrate the skin after physical activity

= precautions: Use in moderation due to the menthol content; avoid topical application during pregnancy; not to be used topically by people who are hyperactive or experience epilepsy or convulsions; highly stimulating, do not use before sleep; store away from homeopathic remedies; do not take orally; keep out of reach of children; follow directions for use and dosage recommendations; for adult use only

= Peppermint oil aids recovery. It is a stimulating oil and promotes a sense of general wellbeing. It also promotes clear thinking, activates the mind and assists with the assimilation of information. Use it to kick start the intellect and process new ideas and concepts.

Use as a digestive aid. Also, with its antispasmodic and analgesic qualities, peppermint helps relieve nerve pain such as sciatica and toothache.

Inhaled directly from the bottle, it clears the head and works as an effective treatment for travel sickness, nausea and sinusitis. As a mild expectorant, it's also good for chest and intestinal disorders. In steam inhalation, peppermint oil can bring immediate relief to sinus congestion, clearing the head and nasal passages.

# Rose

- = **key** words: Passionate, feminine and alluring
- = **botanical** name: *Rosa damascena*
- = **countries** of origin: Bulgaria, Turkey and Iran
- = **derived** from: The flower
- = **blends well** with: Bergamot, Roman chamomile, clary sage, frankincense, geranium, jasmine, lavender, marjoram, neroli, patchouli, rosemary, rosewood, sandalwood and ylang ylang
- = virtues: Gives courage to deal with broken hearts, depression, anxiety, jealousy, resentment, anger, grief; helps reduce symptoms of liver disorders; alleviates hangovers; reduces inflammation and circulatory disturbances; may treat symptoms of menopause, frigidity, uterine imbalance, painful periods, excessive bleeding; helps broken capillaries, rashes, boils, dry and dehydrated skin
- = skin care: Helps balance the skin, especially dry, mature and wrinkled skin; beneficial for inflammation and swelling; regenerates and rehydrates cells; strengthens capillaries; and soothes the skin

= precautions: Avoid on hypersensitive skin; avoid topical application during pregnancy; do not take orally; keep out of reach
of children; follow directions for use and dosage recommendations

= Rose is an emmenagogue, which means it helps menstrual flow.
It also helps to regulate menstruation and relieve the symptoms of
PMS. Rose is also an impressive liver and spleen tonic; it stimulates
bile secretion and purifies the blood.

A splendid antidepressant and superb treatment for grief, rose oil
helps to balance the emotions. Rose is regarded as the 'healer of the
heart'; it relieves mental anguish and emotional turmoil associated
with grief, anger (at self or others), jealousy or resentment.

Also useful as a skin toner for every skin type; particularly good
in the treatment of dryness associated with mature skin. It can also
be used as a treatment for postnatal depression.

# Rosemary

= **key** words: Awakening, exhilarating and builds confidence

= **botanical** name: *Rosmarinus officinalis*

= **countries** of origin: Spain, Tunisia and Morocco

= **derived** from: The herb

= **blends well** with: Basil, bergamot, cedarwood, eucalyptus, frankincense, grapefruit, lemon, lemongrass, lime, peppermint, rose, tea tree

= virtues: Improves concentration and recall while it relieves mental fatigue, tiredness, poor memory, lethargy and drowsiness; improves concentration and will; aids poor circulation; helps relieve the symptoms of back pain, as well as muscular aches and pains; helps relieve rheumatic cramps, gout, sprains, obesity, liver congestion; helps treat alopecia (baldness) and headaches

= skin care: Regenerates cells; strengthens saggy skin; reduces water retention; strengthens and stimulates hair growth; adds lustre to hair; treats oily hair and dandruff

= precautions: To be used with extreme caution with people who have epilepsy and high blood pressure; avoid topical application during pregnancy; may cause irritation on sensitive or damaged skin; highly stimulating, do not use before sleep or with people who are hyperactive; do not take orally; keep out of reach of children; follow directions for use and dosage recommendations

= In ancient times, rosemary was used for memory and is still known today as one of the most stimulating and awakening essential oils. Its strongest effect is on the nervous system. As an oil which heightens sensory perception and stimulates recall, it can act as a brain stimulant. Simply inhale a few drops to keep focused and allay any worries.

Rosemary oil promotes confidence and can help people with low self-esteem. It also helps tired or injured muscles recuperate, and due to its effect on the circulatory system, it is useful for rheumatic cramps and assists any area of the body that lacks mobility. With its stimulating effect, it helps cleanse and detoxify the body and so alleviates liver congestion.

Also good for hair care, leaving hair radiant with a rich lustre. Can also stimulate hair growth.

# Rosewood

- = **key** words: Restoring, hydrating and caring
- = **botanical** name: *Aniba roseodora*
- = **countries** of origin: Various districts of Brazil
- = **derived** from: The wood
- = **blends well** with: Basil, Roman chamomile, cedarwood, geranium, jasmine, lavender, mandarin, marjoram, orange, patchouli, rose, sandalwood and ylang ylang
- = virtues: A good stabilizer for emotional extremes exacerbated by stress and tension; helps relieve headaches and soothe a restless mind; helps dismiss uneasiness; treats infection, parasites, flu, coughs, sore throats, nausea and bronchial disorders; aged and tired skin; reduces jetlag and weariness; improves general wellbeing
- = skin care: Soothes and supports aged and tired skin; heals; treats scars, acne, dry and sensitive skin including eczema and psoriasis; restores elasticity; rejuvenates tired skin
- = precautions:: May cause dermatitis and skin reactions on highly sensitive skin types; avoid topical application during the first three

months of pregnancy; do not take orally; keep out of reach of children; follow directions for use and dosage recommendations

= Rosewood oil inspires a sense of wellbeing and restfulness as it eases the mind. It is a wonderful oil for quiet moments. Especially beneficial during times of grief and bereavement as it brings emotional peace to a wounded heart. It can warm the body and restore connections with loved ones. It can also be effective in the bedroom to inspire intimacy and sensuality.

Rosewood oil helps to release tension, especially for people who suffer headaches due to concentrated activity. It brings ease to difficult times as it releases stress from the body and mind. Soaking in an aromatic bath of rosewood is the perfect end to a stressful day.

With its antibacterial properties, rosewood promotes the body's own natural defence systems, and as a general tonic it helps maintain balance. Applied to the chest, a combination of rosewood, lavender and marjoram essential oils will help relieve spasmodic coughing during flu and colds. It is also an excellent cell regenerator.

# Sandalwood

- = **key** words: Perseverance, tenacity and courage
- = **botanical** name: *Santalum album* and *Santalum spicatum*
- = **countries** of origin: India, Indonesia and Australia
- = **derived** from: The twig
- = **blends well** with: Bergamot, cedarwood, clary sage, frankincense, geranium, jasmine, lavender, mandarin, marjoram, neroli, orange, rose, rosewood, ylang ylang
- = virtues: Helps people face isolation, aggressive and obsessive behaviour, insecurity, possessiveness, nightmares, fear and depression; helps treat genito-urinary problems – cystitis, urinary tract infections, kidney disorders

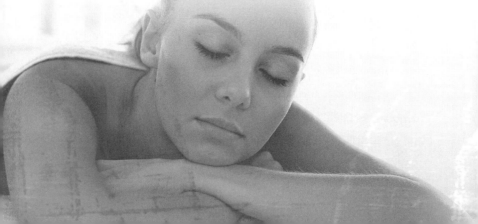

- = skin care: Promotes elasticity; soothes and has anti-inflammatory actions; helps heal itchy skin and inflamed conditions such as eczema and psoriasis; helps acne and dry and chaffed skin; excellent aftershave and moisturiser; heals
- = precautions: Avoid topical application during first three months of pregnancy; do not take orally; keep out of reach of children; follow directions for use and dosage recommendations

= Sandalwood is a strengthening oil, as it promotes courage and releases irrational fear. It can have a stabilising influence during times of dramatic change, and has long been used in prayer, meditation and ritual because it brings harmony to mind, body and spirit.

Sandalwood's cooling and healing properties make it an excellent oil for genito-urinary disorders. In Ayurvedic practices, its anti-inflammatory and anti-infectious properties help to treat 'hot' conditions in the body such as inflammation, irritation and infection.

When the two species of sandalwood are blended they have far greater antibacterial qualities, enhancing the performance of this oil.

# Tea Tree

= **key** words: Clearing, oxygenating and responsive

= **botanical** name: *Melaleuca alternifolia*

= **countries** of origin: Various districts in Australia

= **derived** from: The leaves

= **blends well** with: Bergamot, cedarwood, eucalyptus, frankincense, grapefruit, lavender, lemon, lemongrass, lime, peppermint, rosemary

= **virtues**: Helps counteract feelings of victimisation, deep depression, low morale, fatigue; its anti-fungal properties assist with thrush, Athlete's foot, ringworm, cold sores and respiratory disorders such as asthma, coughs, colds and flu; treats viruses, cysts, boils, acne, open wounds, bacterial infections, low resistance, chronic ill health, recurring infections and poor circulation

= **skin care**: Cleanses, disinfects; treats acne and abscesses; soothes herpes; reduces dandruff; good for oily skin, rashes, warts and ringworm

= precautions: Possible irritant on highly sensitive skin; keep away from eyes; keep away from children; avoid topical application during pregnancy; store away from homeopathic remedies; do not take orally; keep out of reach of children; follow directions for use and dosage recommendations

= Tea tree oil has many uses and is a powerful anti-bacterial, anti-viral and anti-fungal. When the body is threatened, tea tree increases its ability to respond and resist. It was traditionally used in the Australian outback as a medicine for coughs and colds.

We can become vulnerable to infections when we are feeling despondent or in low spirits. Tea tree acts as an energetic pick-me-up and at the same time builds resistance and protection. It's a booster physically and emotionally.

Tea tree acts quickly to eradicate harmful organisms in the body and prevent further infection. It is effective against bites, stings, boils, thrush, sore throats, sinusitis, cuts and grazes, truly first aid in a bottle. It is also an excellent skin toner and works especially well on oily or infected skin to cleanse and disinfect.

# Ylang ylang

= **key** words: Sensuality, intimacy and tenderness

= **botanical** name: *Cananga odorata*

= **countries** of origin: Comoros Islands (off the coast of North Africa), Madagascar and Philippines

= **derived** from: The flower

= **blends well** with: Bergamot, cedarwood, clary sage, jasmine, lavender, mandarin, neroli, orange, patchouli, rose, rosewood, and sandalwood

= virtues: Useful for emotional frigidity, depression, anxiety, frustration, anger, guilt, jealousy, resentment; may assist in the treatment of heart irregularities: Racing heart, palpitations and hypertension; promotes sexual expression; reduces muscular cramps and spasms; used in the treatment of epilepsy

= skin care: Balances the skin; treats dry, oily and combination skin; relieves insect bites; excellent hair tonic for a dry scalp; balances sebum production

= precautions: Can cause headiness in high doses; do not use topically on inflamed, sensitive or reddened skin; avoid topical application during the first three months of pregnancy; do not take orally; keep out of reach of children; follow directions for use and dosage recommendations

= Ylang ylang oil helps uplift the spirits and dissolve resentment. Its warming qualities promote sensuality and encourage physical intimacy as it has the capacity to dismiss emotional frigidity.

If feeling disassociated, soak in an aromatic bath of ylang ylang oil to please and arouse the senses. The oil has the ability to calm and support, and it reduces hyperactivity, palpitations and blood pressure. It is distinctive in its ability to act as a powerful antidepressant, and is extremely effective in the treatment of anxiety, anger and hysterical states.

chapter 5

## home **spa** treatments

Many of the things we do every day have a singular function and can become mundane and routine, taking a shower or bath for example. But now that you've equipped yourself in preparation for your *home spa* you can transform a routine experience into a multifunctional opportunity, one that nurtures and pampers you. For example, if you fill a 100ml bottle with purified water and add two drops of sandalwood, you can spray your hair before you brush it and so condition it and add shine. The same blend can double as an aftershave, perfume or room spray. Or add four to five drops in total of rosemary, bergamot and frankincense to a large stainless steel or glass bowl filled with warm water. This becomes your footbath, as you recline in front of the TV, sit at the dinner table or work at your desk, to relieve tired, sore feet and help dispel stress. Or enjoy a relaxing or energizing start to your day by simply adding five drops of essential oil (in total) onto the floor of your shower recess, perhaps lime, lemon and rosemary, and cover the plug with a wet face cloth. Turn on the hot tap to release the vapours and breathe deeply as you adjust the water and climb in. Your feet will receive a treatment, too. Every moment of your life is an opportunity for enhanced pleasure, a chance to further heal and nurture yourself.

One of the most effective ways to benefit from the use of essential oils is to dilute them in a fragrant free daily body oil. In this way, you create your own individual aromatherapy blend to rub into your skin as the ultimate moisturizer. And the best way to rub it into your skin is with massage. So let's begin our spa treatments with a pleasurable self-massage.

(Heat and water can enhance the permeability of essential oils. For example, lavender is absorbed much quicker when the skin is still damp, and if you warm the surface of your skin with brisk hand movements, you dilate the pores and speed the transfer of essential oils into your skin.)

# massage *magic*

In today's busy world we seem to have no trouble filling our time with things to do. Yet few of us leave enough time to touch or to be touched in day-to-day life. We receive more sensory stimulation through sight and sound than through the sensation of touch. Yet the skin (and the underlying tissue and organs) benefits when it's stroked and caressed with attentive care, so let's not waste another minute.

Self-massage is the perfect way to start your day and it only need take a few minutes. It's best to do it as part of your morning program. And if you like to take a shower in the morning, do it immediately after that. It's as easy as moisturizing your skin.

First, choose an aromatherapy blend that has already been prepared by yourself or an aromatherapist. The secret to optimum health is to keep your body guessing. I therefore suggest you rotate your blends daily. To make your own blend, you will need a fragrance-free daily body oil to use as a base. Then you add your selection of essential oils to the base oil. Following is the recommended dosage for massage (topical application):

✓ Sixteen years to adult: The ratio of essential oils to base oil (such as a blend of either sweet almond, peach kernel, macadamia nut, jojoba, evening primrose or rosehip) should be 1:2. In other words, five drops of essential oil for every 10mls of base oil.

✓ Birth to two years: As a general rule it is recommended to avoid using essential oil blends on the skin unless treating a specific physiological imbalance. The preparation should be highly diluted: One drop in total of essential oil for every 10mls of base oil and applied once a day for a three-day period only. Instead of massage, rely on the other methods of use to calm infants, such as vaporization, compress or bath.

✓ Five to ten years: Make a blend using two drops in total of essential oil for every 10mls of base oil.

✓ Ten to sixteen years: Make a blend using 4 drops of essential oil in total for every 10mls of base oil.

To make an informed selection of three or four essential oils you'd like to add to the base oil, refer to Chapter 4 or rely on your intuition to choose which oils you want to add. It is easy to change your essential oil blend daily when you make a small amount. And it's important to avoid familiarity, as a blend that is great for your body, mind and emotions one day may not be appropriate the next. Every day is different, and with aromatherapy we are able to address our ever-changing physiological and psychological needs.

## massage tips to *remember*:

- ✓ Keep your room and body warm as your body temperature drops as you relax.
- ✓ Create a clean, tidy and warm space to do the massage.
- ✓ Make sure you're comfortable. Use a pillow as a prop to alleviate pressure under ankles, knees, chest or belly.
- ✓ Watch your posture. Keep a straight back and don't put undue pressure on your joints. If you're kneeling, support your knees by resting on a cushion.
- ✓ To apply the oil dip the fingers of one hand into the blend. Rub hands together to spread the oil over the surface of both hands before you apply it to your body.
- ✓ Keep as much of the entire surface of your hand on the skin as you can. Start with the back.
- ✓ Make sure that when you apply pressure to the limbs that it is in the direction of the heart. In that way you work with the blood and lymph flow.

Now you need to know a few good self-massage strokes.

## effleurage

It is easy to practise these moves when you're seated. Allow the flat of your hand to take the shape of your body. Face your fingertips towards each other so that the middle fingers nearly meet. Effleurage (also known as the rowing stroke) consists of long, light movements which prepare the skin for deeper touch. Start at the bottom of the spine (the tips of the fingers of both hands should be placed on the bottom of the spine) and slowly move up the back applying firm pressure to the sides of the spine rather than the spine itself. Rotate the fingertips up and outward to move over the shoulders blades (or as far as you can reach), then draw each hand down the sides of the body to begin at the base again. You can also practice this technique on your thigh: Start at the top of the leg and move toward the knee.

Use the effleurage stroke at the start and end of a massage as it calms, relaxes, warms the muscles and stimulates the circulation of blood. The movement should be slow and gentle and the strokes broad so they cover as much of the skin as possible. A blend of lavender, mandarin and ylang ylang will enhance the overall effects of this movement.

## petrissage or *kneading*

Imagine you're kneading dough. This is a more energetic movement: Lift and squeeze the muscles (don't pinch) with the hands. Take hold of the flesh between thumb and fingers and pull it away from the bone; knead it. It encourages the flow of nutrients and pumps away built-up toxins and wastes. It also promotes blood flow and releases stress. The shoulders, neck and buttocks (areas where we store stress) greatly benefit from the petrissage stroke. A blend of lavender, bergamot and cedarwood can help reduce anxiety.

## *friction*

Use friction to concentrate on one area of tension. On small areas of the body, such as the base (sacrum) of the spine, it is usually carried out with the soft cushion of the thumbs or fingers, though the strokes can be done with the heel or entire flat surface of the hand on large areas. The part of the hand in contact with the skin should move quickly and lightly as a warm up stroke. This is especially good when applying a blend over the spine. (A blend of eucalyptus, lemon and tea tree is great for respiratory conditions such as bronchitis, flu or cold.) Deeper friction can be applied using slow, deep, circular movements, and is ideal for the feet or lower back. Relieve muscular pain with a blend of rosemary, eucalyptus and lemongrass. Friction helps break down fibrous knots and tension nodules, and increases peripheral circulation.

## tapotement or *percussion*

Percussion strokes work effectively as an expectorant and are great for any one who has trouble breathing or a mucousy chest infection. A blend of eucalyptus, peppermint, tea tree and lemon will work wonders. The stroke is essentially a rapid slapping action using cupped hands. Cup your hands then with palms down chop along the fleshy parts of the body (not too rigorously). Practise on your thigh; it should sound like a galloping horse. This helps stimulate or relax the respiratory system, circulation and nerves (depending on your essential oil blend) and at the same time helps release mucus. It is said to improve muscle tone and firm slackened skin, but that depends on the length of time and regularity that it is performed. It is best used along the backs of the legs and the upper back (be careful over the kidney area). The effectiveness of the stroke depends on quick successive movements performed without breaking the rhythm.

## do not *massage*

×     If you have an infection, a high temperature, a fever or a disease. Check with your doctor first.

×     After recent surgery, broken bones, if you have an open wound or swelling or directly over a healing site.

×     During skin eruptions such as severe acne, a skin disease, eczema or a rash.

×     If you have a heart condition, varicose veins or other chronic circulatory problems.

×     A history of back problems or acute back pain.

×     On the first day of menstruation.

×     If you have had recent inoculations.

×     Straight after a heavy meal. You should allow two hours to digest before a massage.

Massage stirs lymph and blood flow, so it can spread infection and overwhelm the nervous system. Gentle rubbing or stroking may relieve back pain, but only qualified professionals should exert pressure on bones, joints, the spine or on weak or sore backs. Under these conditions, simply give or receive a hand or foot massage as a safe, nurturing alternative.

## massage & *pregnancy*

It is important to keep your skin moisturised and supple during pregnancy to help prevent stretch marks. I recommend an enriching blend of jojoba, evening primrose and rosehip oils. Massage both the nipples (to toughen them for breast feeding) and the perineum (to prepare for birth). Avoid all essential oils on the skin during the first three months of pregnancy, and thereafter one weekly aromatherapy self-massage is enough. Focus on your legs, arms, head, feet and back. Always follow the guidelines in the essential oil compendium (Chapter 4) before you self-treat with essential oils. And when you are pregnant, it's best to check with a doctor or qualified practitioner before you begin.

You can still vaporize, compress, inhale, shower and bathe with essential oils. It's only the topical application that you need to be careful with. During pregnancy, please avoid the topical application of the following essential oils: Basil, clary sage, cedarwood, cypress, eucalyptus, lemongrass, lime, fennel, frankincense, ginger, marjoram, peppermint, rosemary, rose, sage, tea tree and thyme.

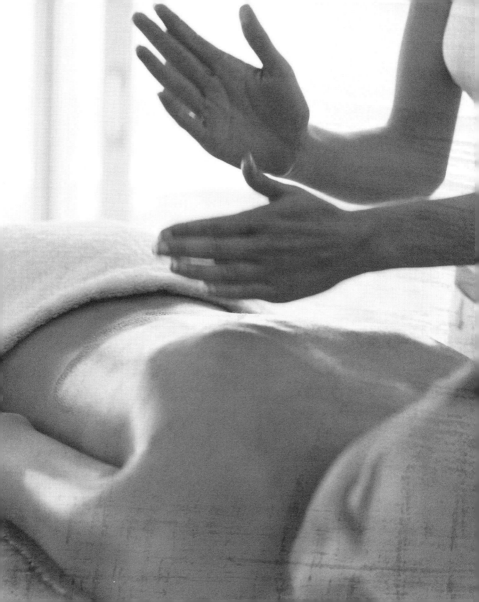

# the beauty of a *bath*

Your bathroom is transformed into a mini-spa the moment you put your essential oils out on the bench. (Note the word *bench*, rather than cupboard. If your oils are out of sight, they are usually out of mind.)

The bath is one of the best places to de-stress when you use your tub as a treatment space rather than simply a washing place. Any time when you need ten minutes for quiet reflection, do it in the privacy of your tub. You can set the scene with a candle.

Use a total of three to six drops of essential oil in the bath. Halve the dosage for children and halve again for infants. Once you've turned the taps off, agitate the surface of the water. Swish it rigorously to disperse the molecules. You'll notice a tiny aromatic film float on the surface and coat your skin as you lower yourself into the tub. The oil molecules hover in the air for more than 15 minutes as they evaporate, though your nose can no longer detect the smell after a few minutes as odour fatigue sets in. Don't be tempted to add more oils to the bath. The oils continue to work long after you can no longer detect any smell. When it comes to the potency of an essential oil bath, less is more. Use your intuition as well as your sense of smell to determine which oils to add to your bath, and don't forget to refer to the compendium (Chapter 4) if you have a specific concern you would like to address.

# scentual *showers*

For a sensual aromatic shower experience, you first need to place a wet facecloth over the plughole. Sprinkle five drops (in total) of your chosen essential oils onto the shower recess: Lime, lemon and rosemary will awaken and focus the mind, and eucalyptus, tea tree and lemongrass are good if you're especially tired and lethargic. Use a blend of rosewood, cedarwood and lavender if you have been feeling acutely stressed and overwhelmed. Turn on the hot tap. The moment the water hits the essential oils, the molecules rise and disperse and all you have to do is breathe deeply. Adjust the taps to warm and step in.

The antiseptic, antiviral and antibacterial qualities of essential oils also provide your feet with a treat. Say goodbye to fungal infections and hello to improved circulation (add bergamot to treat foot odour).

After a few minutes, pick up the aromatic facecloth and sponge it over your skin. Wring it out and wash your face. The essential oils now become a first-aid treatment for your face and body. Water helps essential oils to absorb more easily into the skin and when they're inhaled with every breath, they help soothe the body and soul simultaneously.

# aromatic *vapours*

Vaporizing essential oils is one of the most effective ways to inspire psychological wellbeing. The fragrant molecules of the essential oils help disinfect the air, and they also help lift your mood and sharpen your mind and senses.

When asked which is the best way to infuse essential oils, I generally recommend the Aromamist battery operated vaporizer as it works to a timer and requires no electricity, candles or maintenance. Electric vaporizers are great too because they're effective and safe around the elderly and children. If you use a candle for your vaporizer, then choose beeswax nightlight candles, as they are better for your health and the environment.

You can use essential oils in a vaporizer to reduce airborne bacteria, to enhance memory and focus as you study, to expand creative flair, to induce sleep or to create your personal ambience. You can also vaporize essential oils to enhance romance and intimacy. It is the easiest way to instantly create a mini-spa environment anywhere in your home to nurture and heal. Check the essential oil compendium (Chapter 4) to help you pick the best essential oils combinations to vaporize for any occasion.

# quick *pick-me-ups*

Never miss an opportunity to enhance your health and wellness; recharge mundane or routine activities with essential oils. Every time you are at your bathroom basin – even if it's to clean your teeth – seize a moment to de-stress. Put the plug in, run hot water until the basin is half full and add three to four drops of your chosen essential oil. Agitate the water, grab a towel and place it over your head, then bend over the basin (keep your head approximately eight inches from the surface), close your eyes and breathe deeply in and out.

With this simple pick-me-up spa treatment, you can help relieve a range of conditions such as mental fatigue (basil, mandarin and lavender); worry (bergamot, lavender and geranium); anxiety and depression (clary sage, orange and bergamot); the symptoms of a head cold (lemon, tea tree and eucalyptus); and sinus congestion (peppermint and eucalyptus). The warm water gently steams your skin, cleanses and releases toxins and encourages a glowing complexion.

# aromatic *first aid*

Essential oil compresses make perfect first aid treatments. Apply a compress to relieve the pain and swelling of a bite or wound, as it can help speed recovery. A compress can also be used to relieve painful arthritic joints, stomach pain, headaches, sprains, varicose veins and sore muscles.

A compress can be cold or hot; it depends on the type of injury or pain. Hot compresses are most often used to treat chronic pain, and cold compresses are used to treat acute pain such as a first aid for injuries such as sprains. Insect bites are usually treated with a cold compress because heat can spread the poison, and period pain and arthritis are better treated with a warm compress.

You can also use an essential oil compress as a gentle way to exfoliate dead skin cells and restore a healthy glow to facial skin. It's as easy as adding three drops in total of your favourite oil into a basin or bowl filled with water. (Agitate the surface before you immerse the face cloth.) As a treatment for your face, a compress is beneficial for the treatment of acne, pimples or enlarged dirty pores (especially if you smoke cigarettes), or you can use a (hot) compress to soften the bristles of a beard before shaving.

To apply your compress, wring it out slowly until it stops dripping, though with ample water still left on the cloth. Open it out flat over your palms and apply to your skin using a press and release action. Repeat this process three times to help the lymphatic system cleanse any impurities.

A few other points:

- ✓ Hot compresses are particularly helpful for the treatment of backache, period pain, rheumatic and arthritic pain, earache and toothache.
- ✓ Cold compresses are helpful for the treatment of headaches, sprains, tennis elbow and other 'hot' inflamed or swollen conditions.
- ✓ Hot compresses dilate or open the blood vessels and bring more blood to the area. Cold compresses constrict or shrink the blood supply. By alternating hot and cold compresses, you can help stabilise some injuries and drain excess fluid and toxins from the area. This technique may be useful in the treatment of sprains or sore muscles after a rigorous workout. Always start with a hot compress and finish with a cold one.

✓ Do not apply a compress to an infant or children up to two years of age, or several compresses over large areas of the body.

## aromatic footbath

If you are able to sit in one spot for more than five minutes, then you can give your feet a treat, an aromatic footbath. Simply get a large bowl (large enough to fit your feet comfortably), fill it half full with very warm water, add five drops of essential oil and agitate the surface of the water. It's that simple. And it not only relaxes, it improves circulation, protects feet from fungal infections, strengthens nails, softens skin and relaxes muscles and tendons. Keep a hand towel close by so you can dry your feet after you're done. This is a deeply relaxing mini-spa treat for feet. Refer to the compendium of essential oils (Chapter 4) if you want to treat a specific ailment, or create a particular mood.

(If you have the time, you can also give the bottoms of your feet a good scrub with a pumice stone to remove hard, dead skin, or you may want to wait until your next aromatic bath.)

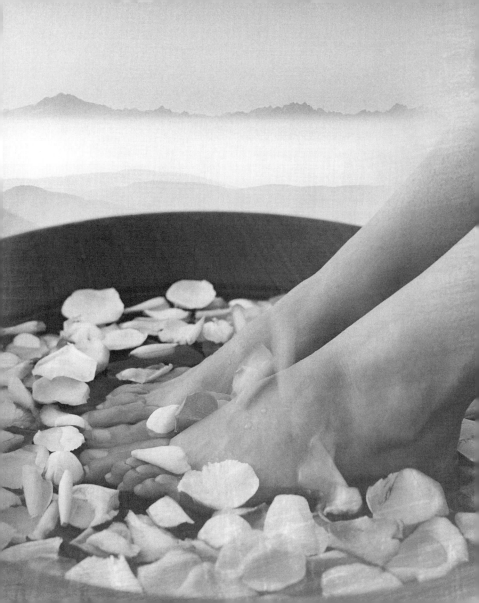

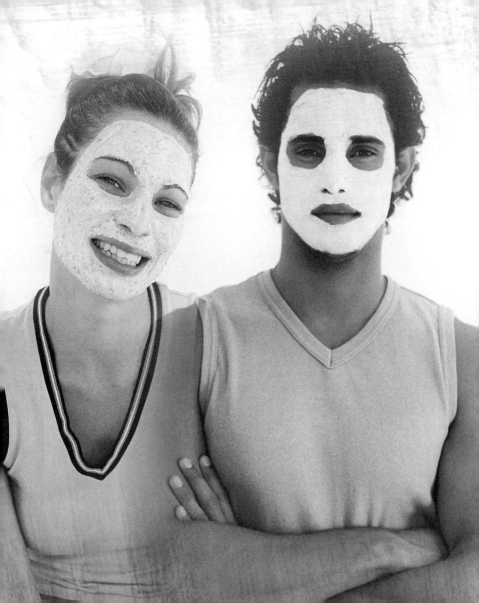

# deluxe aromatherapy facial & scalp *treatment*

A facial is a sensual spa treatment. It is a great way to relax as well as an effective treatment for you skin. You can use essential oils to help oily and acne prone skin, dry and mature skin and sensitive skin. Check the essential oil compendium (Chapter 4) to see which oils best suit your skin type.

The following do-it-yourself facial and scalp treatment is the perfect gift you can give yourself. I suggest you record the instructions onto a tape recorder before you begin so you won't need to stop halfway through the treatment to see what comes next. To start you will need a natural bristle brush (the bristles stimulate your scalp) and your favourite facial oil. Simply add one drop of essential oil into a daily body oil especially designed for a facial treatment. An ideal combination is jojoba, evening primrose and rosehip oils. There are excellent essential oil facial blends available (pre-blended for your convenience) that include rose, jasmine, neroli, lavender or Roman chamomile (check the compendium to determine which best suits your skin type).

Now you're ready to begin:

✓ Sit comfortably in a straight-back chair, uncross your feet and place them flat on the floor. Take a deep breath and release a big sigh. Place your open hands onto your lap face down. Close your eyes and gently raise the tip of your tongue to the roof of your mouth. Begin to take deep, slow rhythmic breaths in and out of your nose.

✓ Run your hands up your thigh, over your tummy, up and over your chest, up and over either side of your throat and onto the top of head. Imagine that an egg has broken on the top of your skull, open your fingers and gently and slowly run them down over your entire face. It should feel as though the egg white is running over your skin.

✓ Keep your eyes closed and draw your hands down over your eyes so that your palm covers your entire eye socket. Keep your fingers together and breathe in and out slowly and deeply through the nose.

✓ Slide the fingers down so they sit across the top of each eyebrow. Use your fingertips and press strongly into the sinus area at the (inner) tip of each eyebrow; slide your fingers outward (use a press and release action) to the outer edge of each eyebrow. Repeat three times. Now move under the eyebrow and press up and into the skull with the same press and release action; again slide across the length of each eyebrow toward the outer edge. Repeat three times.

Now slide the fingers gently inward over your closed eyelid until the middle finger finds that tiny spot near the corner of your eye next to your nose. Take a moment to press and release the middle finger into that spot. Repeat three times.

✓ With one hand, pinch either side of your nose with your thumb and forefinger; press and release. Repeat three times. Glide your fingers down under your cheekbone and move outward towards the outer side of your face: Your fingers should still be under your cheekbone and in line with your temples. With the pads of your fingers pressed in deeply, move them in a forward circular direction three times and then backwards in a circular direction three times. It is here (the temporomandibular joint or jaw bone) where most facial tension occurs and is stored. When we feel our ability to communicate is blocked, this area can become tender and tight. This simple massage with your facial oil will help bring relief.

✓ Move both hands out towards the ears, and with your thumb and the side of your forefinger squeeze and roll the ear lobe, up to the top of the ear and down again. Now place each thumb in each ear over the ear hole to close off any sound. Breathe in and out through the nose deeply. Repeat three times.

Expand your lungs more with every breath you take. Complete with a massage of the entire inner and outer surface of your ears with your thumbs and fingers.

✓ Move the pads of your fingers back onto the cheeks and allow the jaw to drop open. Massage the entire cheek area; move the skin over the bone in a circular action upward and out-ward. With your fingertips faced towards each other, place them over your lips. Your forefinger will sit above your lips, your middle finger will sit on your lips and your ring finger will sit below your lips. Draw both hands simultaneously and slowly upward and outward towards the ears. Then remove your hands from your face, replace them on your lips and repeat the stroke… and again for a third time.

✓ Move both hands to the centre of your chin. Your finger-tips will sit on the soft tissue of the chin with your thumbs underneath it. Draw and squeeze the skin in-between the fingers and thumbs. Move up the chin towards the ears. Repeat three times.

✓ Slide your fingers to the base of your neck and massage deeply into the shoulders. Allow your elbows to fall naturally onto your chest as you do this.

✓ Use a circular motion on either side of the spine and work up towards the base of the skull. Press deeply into the base of the skull as you move towards the ears. Repeat three times.

✓ As though you were shampooing your hair, move your fingers back and forward over the entire surface of the skull. Begin in the centre and move outward in a back and forward motion. Repeat several times.

✓ With a natural bristle brush, comb over the entire surface of you scalp rigorously. This is an excellent technique to stimulate blood flow to the area. It will help reduce hair loss and improve the condition of the skin, especially for people prone to dandruff, eczema or psoriasis.

✓ Return your fingers to the top of your head. Spread your forefingers and thumb and gently repeat the egg white stroke as described above. Run your fingers over your face, down your throat, over your chest and abdominal area to your thighs. Breathe deeply in and slowly out through your nose three times.

✓ Allow your head to stretch over toward the right hand shoulder. Hold the position for a few seconds then slowly return your head to centre. Then take your head to the left hand shoulder, as you did the right. Hold the stretch for several seconds then slowly return to centre. Now allow your head to drop forward to your chest as far as you can comfortably go. Hold for several seconds then return your head to centre. Next allow your head to drop backwards to stretch out the entire throat region. When you go as far as you comfortably can, stay there for several seconds and then slowly return your head to centre.

✓ Shrug your shoulders up towards your ears, hold for a moment and relax. Repeat three times. Then lift and rotate your shoulders backwards in a circular direction three times. Then repeat three times in a forward circular motion.

✓ Sit still and in your own time slowly open your eyes. You're done.

There are many ways to pamper yourself in your home mini-spa, and in addition to the treatments suggested here you're certain to find many other ways to nurture and relax yourself now that your *home spa* is up and on its feet. Read the next chapter for a few more quick and easy *home spa* treatments, and don't forget to take notes and inspiration from your monthly or bi-monthly spa visits.

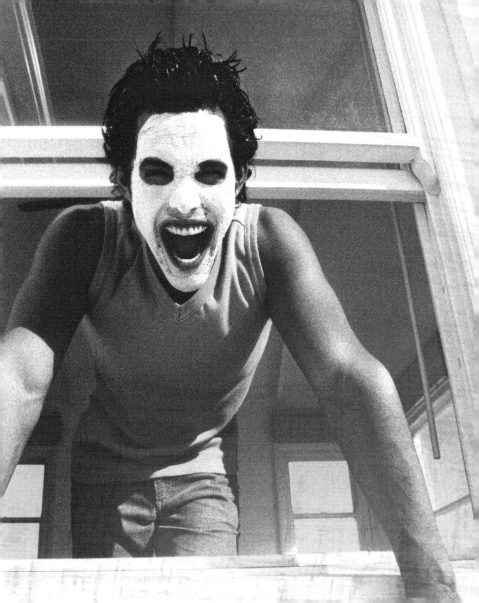

chapter 6

## 28-day **refocus** program

If you like the idea of having a mini-spa environment at home, yet
don't think you have the time to enjoy it, try the 28-Day Refocus program. It's intended to show you that with *home spa* you can nurture
yourself in some tiny way at least daily. It takes 28 days to create a
habit, so after you've completed the program, I'm certain you'll continue to find the time every day to care for yourself in some small
way. And you can return to the program for inspiration at any time,
particularly if you feel stuck; that is, you know you want to do something good for yourself but you don't know exactly what.

Remember to improvise if you don't have something you need. If
you don't have a bath, take an aromatic shower; if you don't have a recommended oil, then use what you have. If you don't have a vaporizer,

make one: Take a bowl and fill it with close to boiling water and add a few drops of essential oil (remember to keep it in a safe place away from children). If you don't have a spray bottle to spritz with aromatic water, then make the aromatic water in the bowl, dip in a fork and flick it onto your sheets or onto the liner of your drawers. It's easy to improvise, so let's go.

(I've included the Two-Minute Body Rub – which can certainly be longer if you have the time – regularly in the 28-Day Refocus Program as I think it's one of the most simple and effective *home spa* treatments that you could give yourself, and I hope that the Program inspires you to incorporate it into your life daily.)

## *day* 1: mini aroma bath

✓ Take a quick three-minute aromatherapy sponge bath before going to bed: Fill the tub with just a few inches of water, add three drops of essential oil in total and agitate the surface. Then step into the bath and with a face cloth, sponge your body. Try lavender, marjoram and sandalwood as a blend. You'll find it's a great way to help you sleep peacefully.

# *day* 2: vaporize

✓ Vaporize a blend of your favourite essential oils to create an environment that nurtures and heals. Try an energizing combination of bergamot, lime and rosemary or grapefruit as a blend. Use six to eight drops in total.

# *day* 3: two-minute body rub

✓ Moisturise your skin from top to toe with an aromatherapy blend. Choose any two essential oils and add two drops in total to one teaspoon (approximately 5mls) of fragrance free daily body oil or the equivalent amount of an unperfumed body creme. Massage the oil/creme into your skin. (See Massage Magic, Chapter 5.)

# *day* 4: quick pick me-up

✓ Half fill your bathroom basin with hot water and add three drops of essential oil (try eucalyptus to feel more awake and clear headed). Agitate the water. Close your eyes and put your face over the basin with a towel over your head. Draw in three deep breaths.

# day 5: bare feet treat

✓ Find a grassy spot of earth or sand to walk on near your home. Kick off your shoes and socks and walk on the natural earth with bare feet for at lease three minutes. If you are in your garden with fresh petals or herbs, rub the plant on the soles of your feet. Breathe deeply. You can also take the opportunity to anchor your experience to an aroma. When you are in the peak of the experience – full of joy – take the lid off a bottle of essential oil and inhale deeply. In this way, you can link the experience of the moment to the scent you smell.

# day 6: instant pick-me-up

✓ Place one or two drops of essential oil on a handkerchief. Use it throughout the day as an instant pick-me-up: Simply inhale the vapours as you hold the handkerchief over your nostrils. Try lemon, eucalyptus, tea tree or peppermint.

# day 7: compress to go

✓ Immerse a face cloth in aromatic water (fill a bowl with 200ml of water and add three drops in total of essential oil). Wring it out, fold it in half and roll it up. Place it in a small clean plastic bag. Put it in your handbag or briefcase and throughout the day take it out and wipe your face, neck and across your shoulders with it to wipe away any unwanted tension. Especially good in warmer seasons.

# day 8: on the go footsoak

✓ Take the largest bowl you have, fill it with warm water and add five drops of essential oil. Place your feet in the water and relax for 10 minutes, either in silence or as you sit and work, watch TV, read or listen to music. (Make sure you have a bowl at work and home.)

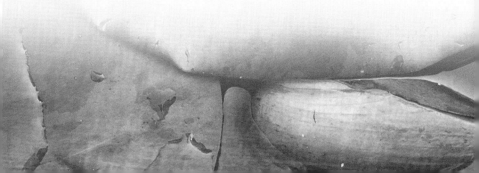

# *day* 9: aromatic sniff

✓ Place a bottle of your favourite essential oil in your handbag or briefcase. Any time you feel stress or strain throughout the day, take out the bottle and have a quick sniff.

# *day* 10: pick-me-up in a cup

✓ Take a favourite essential oil with you to work (peppermint really clears the head). At morning and afternoon tea time, fill a cup with boiling water, add three drops of essential oil and take it back to your desk. While the water remains hot, pick up the cup every now and again and inhale.

# *day* 11: two-minute body rub

✓ Moisturise your skin from top to toe with an aromatherapy blend. Try any two essential oils – make it a different blend to the one you used on Day 3 – and add two drops in total to one teaspoon (approximately 5mls) of fragrance free daily body oil or the equivalent amount of an unperfumed body creme. Massage the oil/creme into your skin. (See Massage Magic, Chapter 5.)

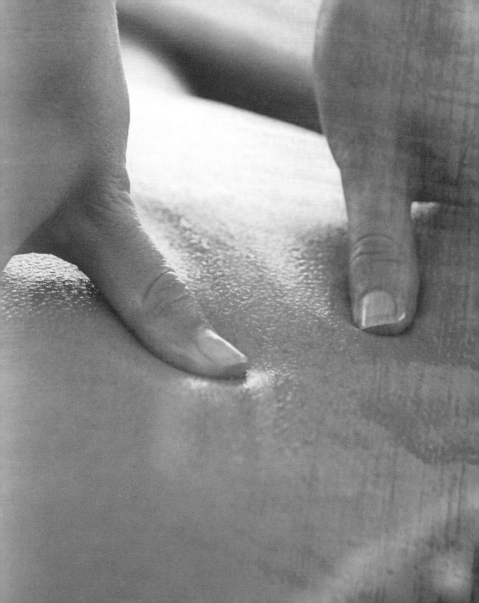

# day 12: synthetic

✓ Make a conscious choice to avoid the use of any synthetic perfumes or products. Make sure that what you put on your skin is pure and natural. Accept that no matter what you have to do today, you can do it naturally. If you must, wear a little lip gloss, but that's it. It is imperative that we own the skin we're in.

# day 13: aromatic shower

✓ Start or end the day with an aromatic shower. Choose up to three of your favourite essential oils, and drop one or two drops of each (five in total) onto the shower recess. Place a wet face cloth over the drain hole in the shower. Turn on the hot tap and wait a few moments for the hot water to release the essential oil molecules. Adjust the taps to the temperature you like, step in and breathe.

# day 14: aromatic hair rinse

✓ Fill an empty glass bottle with water. Add two to three drops (in total) of either rosemary or cedarwood oil, shake well and pour it over your hair as a final rinse in the shower. Leave the aromatic water in your hair. It will treat your hair and scalp and at the same time counteract any anxiety or stress.

## *day* 15: vaporize

✓ Vaporize a blend of your favourite essential oils to create an environment that nurtures and heals. Try a relaxing blend of bergamot, lavender, cedarwood and orange. Use six to eight drops in total.

## *day* 16: two-minute body rub

✓ Moisturise your skin from top to toe with an aromatherapy blend. Choose any two essential oils – make it a different blend to the one you used on Day 11 – and add two drops in total to one teaspoon (approximately 5mls) of fragrance-free daily body oil or the equivalent amount of an unperfumed body creme. Massage the oil/creme into your skin. (See Massage Magic, Chapter 5.)

# day 17: footsoak

✓ Take the largest bowl you have, fill it with warm water and add a few drops of essential oil. Place your feet in the water and relax for 10 minutes, either in silence or as you sit and work, watch TV, read or listen to music. Frankincense is great for fluid retention. (Make sure you have a bowl at work and home.)

# day 18: receive a massage

✓ Book yourself in for a massage. It can be from your partner, a friend or a therapist, whoever is able to care for and nourish you. Make your own aromatherapy blend and take it with you if you like. This is the perfect time to visit a day spa.

# day 19: day's end pick-me-up

✓ As soon as you walk in the door after a day at work, kick off your shoes and peel off your clothes. Go to the bathroom and make a hot aromatic face cloth: Add three drops of your favourite essential oils (in total) to a basin full of warm

water; wet the face cloth in the water then squeeze it out.
Lie down – either on a towel on the bathroom floor or your
bed – and place the cloth over your face. Breathe deeply as
you allow the damp cloth to cool on your skin. Stretch your
arms out as you fill your lungs with the healing vapours.
This only takes a minute or two and is a great way to release
the stress of a super-challenging day.

## day 20: aromatic scrub

✓ Place two tablespoons of salt into a saucer or bowl. Add
three drops of eucalyptus and two drops of tea tree to two
teaspoons of fragrance-free daily body oil – or you can use
olive oil. Pour it over the salt and mix it until blended. Place
it in an easy-to-reach spot near your shower. Climb in and
wet your skin. Turn the taps off and rub the scrub gently over
your skin (not your face). Wash your body as usual. This is a
great exfoliating and detoxifying treatment to do each month.

## day 21: two-minute body rub

✓ Moisturise your body from top to toe with an aromatherapy
blend. Choose any two essential oils – make it a different

blend to the one you used on Day 16 – and add two drops
in total to one teaspoon (approximately 5mls) of fragrance-
free daily body oil or the equivalent amount of an unperfumed body creme. Massage the oil/creme into your skin.
(See Massage Magic, Chapter 5.)

## *day* 22: foot soak

✓ Take the largest bowl you have, fill it with warm water and
add a few drops of essential oil. Choose a different oil from
the one you used on Day 17. Place your feet in the water
and relax for 10 minutes, either in silence or as you watch
TV, read or listen to music.

## *day* 23: two-minute body rub

✓ Moisturise your body from top to toe with an aromatherapy
blend. Choose any two essential oils – make it a different
blend from the one you used on Day 21 – and add two drops
in total to one teaspoon (approximately 5mls) of fragrance-
free daily body oil or the equivalent amount of an unperfumed body creme. Massage the oil/creme into your skin.
(See Massage Magic, Chapter 5.)

# day 24: aromatic drive home

✓ Dispense two to four drops of essential oil onto a tissue and tuck it into the air-conditioning duct of your car. Choose essential oils that will help you stay focused and awake. Rosemary is the most stimulating or try a combination of grapefruit, bergamot, lemon, rosemary and lime.

# day 25: intimacy

✓ Enhance your sensuality and add ylang ylang, orange and patchouli or jasmine to a massage base oil to create a seductive body oil. Rub it into your skin. Then, if possible, offer a sensual massage to your lover or partner.

# day 26: two-minute body rub

✓ Moisturise your body from top to toe with an aromatherapy blend. Choose any two essential oils – make it a different blend to the one you used on Day 23 – and add two drops in total to one teaspoon (approximately 5mls) of fragrance-free daily body oil or the equivalent amount of an unperfumed body creme. Massage the oil/creme into your skin. (See Massage Magic, Chapter 5.)

# *day* 27 : breathe-easy shower

✓ Start the day with a breathe-easy aromatic shower. Choose eucalyptus, peppermint, tea tree and lemon, and drop six drops in total onto the shower recess. Place a wet face cloth over the drain hole in the shower. Turn on the hot tap and wait a few moments for the hot water to release the essential oil molecules. Adjust the taps to the temperature you like, step in and breathe deeply.

# *day* 28 : two-minute body rub

✓ Moisturise your body from top to toe with an aromatherapy blend. Choose any two essential oils – make it a different blend to the one you used on Day 26 – and add two drops in total to one teaspoon (approximately 5mls) of fragrance free daily body oil or the equivalent amount of an unperfumed body creme. Massage the oil/creme into your skin. (See Massage Magic, Chapter 5.)

Nothing ever stays the same, it changes, evolves and transforms. *home spa* inspires you to recognise and accept the nature of change. Every day your body, mind and spirit demands a different sort of treatment than the day before. One day a massage with lavender may be the best medicine, the next a bath with rosewood. The idea is to be in tune with what your body needs and to respond accordingly. I hope my book has assisted in some small way to do that … to know that ultimately you are responsible for your own good health and personal wellbeing and that self-care practices need not be difficult.

## organic and cross cultural essential oils

Purity and quality is paramount to the practice of aromatherapy. Therefore, I personally use my own Organic Aromatherapy and Cross-Cultural Essential Oil range. Each oil is a fusion of certified organic and wild harvest pure essential oils, sourced from the same botanical species gathered from different growing regions around the world. For example, my lavender oil (*lavandula angustifolia*) is sourced from Bulgaria, England, France, Australia, Mongolia and the Ukraine. As a result I've created a lavender oil that is superbly unique, as is the case for every oil in the range. My objective was to create a premium range of essential oils and essential oil blends choosing only the highest grade and quality possible, free from chemicals, pesticides and radiation. I continue to oversee every aspect of production, from hand selecting the ingredients to blending the oil.

Wherever possible, I recommend the use of premium quality organic essential oils for your personal use. Remember to do your homework: Question your essential oil supplier on how it sources its essential oils, how it ensures quality, what grade of oils it purchases and what testing methods it employs to authenticate an oil for its purity and quality.

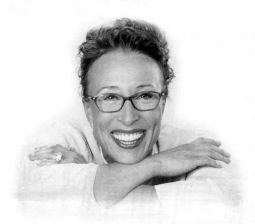

*judith white* is a leading authority on aromatherapy. She has co-authored nine bestselling books on aromatherapy, and continues to pioneer new ways to develop and work with essential oils. Judith appears regularly on television and radio programs, and her inspired work has taught thousands how to use essential oils in a safe and effective way to enhance everyday life.

Judith regularly gives seminars throughout the world and has developed a complete range of aromatherapy and beauty products. For more information, visit **www.judithwhite.com.au** or write to: P.O. Box 12713 A'Beckett Street, Melbourne Victoria Australia 8006.

Notes

# Notes

Notes

Notes

Notes

## Hay House Titles of Related Interest

*Aromatherapy 101,* by Karen Downes

*The Detox Kit,* by Jane Alexander

*Eating in the Light,* by Doreen Virtue, Ph.D.

*Eliminating Stress, Finding Inner Peace* (book-with-CD),
by Brian L. Weiss, M.D.

*Healing with Herbs and Home Remedies A–Z,* by Hanna Kroeger

*Heal Your Body,* by Louise L. Hay

*The Herbal Detox Plan,* by Xandria Williams

*Healthy Body Cards* (a 50-card deck), by Louise L. Hay

*Om Yoga in a Box* (3 separate programs—Basic, Intermediate, and Couples),
by Cyndi Lee

*Shape Your Life,* by Barbara Harris, with Angela Hynes

*The Steps to Healing,* by Dana Ullman, M.P.H.

*Ultimate Pilates,* by Dreas Reyneke

*Vegetarian Meals for People-on-the-Go,* by Vimala Rodgers

*Wheat-Free, Worry-Free,* by Danna Korn

*Yoga Pure and Simple,* by Kisen

All of the above are available at your local bookstore, or may be ordered
by contacting Hay House (see next page).

We hope you enjoyed this Hay House Lifestyles book.
If you would like to receive a free catalogue featuring additional
Hay House books and products, please contact:

P.O. Box 5100
Carlsbad, CA 92018-5100
**(760) 431-7695** or **(800) 654-5126**
**(760) 431-6948 (fax)** or **(800) 650-5115 (fax)**
**www.hayhouse.com**® • **www.hayfoundation.org**

• ◆ •

*Published and distributed in Australia by:* Hay House Australia Pty. Ltd.,
18/36 Ralph St., Alexandria NSW 2015 • *Phone:* 612-9669-4299
*Fax:* 612-9669-4144 • www.hayhouse.com.au

*Published and distributed in the United Kingdom by:* Hay House UK, Ltd.,
292B Kensal Rd., London W10 5BE • *Phone:* 44-20-8962-1230
*Fax:* 44-20-8962-1239 • www.hayhouse.co.uk

*Published and distributed in the Republic of South Africa by:*
Hay House SA (Pty), Ltd., P.O. Box 990, Witkoppen 2068
*Phone/Fax:* 27-11-706-6612 • orders@psdprom.co.za

*Published in India by:* Hay House Publications (India) Pvt. Ltd., Muskaan Complex,
Plot No. 3, B-2, Vasant Kunj, New Delhi 110 070 • *Phone:* 91-11-4176-1620
*Fax:* 91-11-4176-1630 • www.hayhouseindia.co.in

*Distributed in Canada by:* Raincoast, 9050 Shaughnessy St., Vancouver, B.C.
V6P 6E5 • *Phone:* (604) 323-7100 • *Fax:* (604) 323-2600 • www.raincoast.com

• ◆ •

Tune in to **HayHouseRadio.com**® for the best in inspirational talk radio featuring top
Hay House authors! And, sign up via the Hay House USA Website to receive the Hay
House online newsletter and stay informed about what's going on with your favorite
authors. You'll receive bimonthly announcements about Discounts and Offers, Special
Events, Product Highlights, Free Excerpts, Giveaways, and more!
**www.hayhouse.com**®